29 DAYS
... to your perfect weight

A Simple Guide to Permanent Results!

Michele Bertolin
Richard Fast

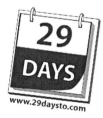

29 DAYS

www.29daysto.com

29 DAYS ... to your perfect weight!

ISBN: 978-0-9865377-1-4

29 DAYS™

1078 Westhaven Drive
Burlington, Ontario
Canada L7P 5B5

www.29daysto.com

Book Design by Janice Phelps, LLC

YOUR SPECIAL 2 DIGIT ISBN NUMBER

Your *29 DAYS* program includes online access to your daily coach.
To gain access to your online coach you will need a special ACCESS
CODE.

To obtain your special ACCESS CODE you will need the last 2 numbers of
your book's ISBN number.

Your 2 DIGIT ISBN number is: 1-4

**TO REGISTER FOR YOUR SPECIAL ACCESS CODE PLEASE GO TO
http://29daysto.com/register/**

A BRIEF OVERVIEW ON HOW THE
29 DAYS COURSES WORK

If you were given a blank canvas and a set of brushes and paints to create a picture, the process of painting would be the same for you as for everyone, but the picture you paint would be uniquely yours. In *29 DAYS* we created a tried and proven process that will work for any number of people, but the discoveries, solutions and results that you uncover, will be as unique to you as your fingerprints.

In just twenty-nine days you will change the way you think! When you think differently, you act and perform differently, and twenty-nine days is all it takes for you to instill lasting, permanent change.

Your life is chock full of habits. Some good, some bad. Imagine what your life would be like if you could get rid of a few habits you don't want or acquire a couple you really do want? What kind of a person would you become? What kind of a life would you enjoy?

- How would you feel if you could become your perfect weight in 29 days?
- How would you feel if you could live the rest of your life without cigarettes in just 29 days?
- Would you like to adopt the habit of learning to save money in just 29 days?
- How about 29 days to become a great listener and communicator?

Humans are generally impatient. When we want a result we want it instantly as in, "Yesterday would be nice; I'll settle for today; and tomorrow is way too late!" In reality, instant results are almost impossible, which means we get side-tracked or bored and soon lose our passion for change. Thus, no change!

29 Days ... to a habit you want!, (a.k.a. "*29 Days*") breaks this self-defeating cycle. It guarantees results and it puts a time stamp on it. Can you wait twenty-nine days for a result that will dramatically change your life forever? If you think you can then this book is for you.

29 Days incorporates the latest technology to help you take control of the greatest asset you have: your thoughts. Here's how it works:

- Read the book *29 DAYS ... to a habit you want!*
- Choose the course that aligns with your desire for change (i.e. Quit Smoking, Lose Weight, become a Great Listener and Communicator etc.)
- Interact with your virtual "online coach" as he guides you, each morning and evening for twenty-nine days, through the necessary steps to permanent change and results.
- After twenty-nine days you will have either acquired a habit you really want, or you will have freed yourself from a habit you desperately want to be rid of.

The ultimate purpose of the *29 DAYS* programs is permanent change. Permanent change can only be achieved by changing your deepest thoughts. You will take small, simple steps that fit into your daily life. In fact, these steps will be so basic and easy, they will naturally and effortlessly become your new lifestyle. That is the *secret* to lasting change!

Change the way you think
and you will change your world.

ACKNOWLEDGMENTS

This book and the associated courses are the result of an enormous amount of effort from a great number of people. I want to express my gratitude and appreciation to:

Michele Bertolin, my wife and my best friend for her tireless guidance and encouragement to get the endless ideas from thought to paper. Michele's efforts in co-writing *29 DAYS... to Your Perfect Weight* speaks for itself. Thanks for always, always being there.

Gavin McDougald who continually donated his time, effort, feedback, and tireless enthusiasm to the myriad of details that are necessary to weave a book, a website and a series of courses into a cohesive whole. Your help, suggestions and guidance from the very beginning made this project possible.

Janice Phelps Williams, for her visual concepts, book design and her editing and re-editing with the patience of Job. Thanks so much for your attention to detail and your invaluable suggestions on improving the *29 DAYS* concept.

Thanks also to Jim Donovan, Janet Cade and Judi Gabai for their encouragement, faith and support for the ideas, format and philosophy of *29 DAYS*.

Then there are all the people who willingly participated as beta testers to ensure the viability, the daily interaction, messaging and overall concept that a twenty-nine day interactive coaching program really works. Your insight, suggestions and daily feedback were vital to creating effective, life-changing programs.

I also wish to thank the collective genius of Zig Ziglar, Maxwell Maltz, Robert Maurer, Jack Canfield, Robert Ringer, Stephen Covey, Mark Victor Hansen, Deepak Chopra, Robert Fritz and Earl Nightingale for their inspiration, writing, philosophy and passion that are so instrumental in making our visit to this planet a better experience.

Book One: *29 DAYS ... to a habit you want!*

Book Two: *29 DAYS ... to your perfect weight*

BOOK ONE

29 DAYS ... to a habit you want!

PREFACE

Behavioral scientists claim that it takes as little as twenty-one days to develop a habit. Is this really true? Maybe ... it all depends on how *you* go about it! If you're going to try to change a habit using willpower, it might as well be twenty-one *years*!

All of us are mirror reflections of our thoughts, fears, beliefs and attitudes. If we cannot change those things, we cannot instill *lasting* results.

> *"We are what we think.*
> *All that we are arises within our thoughts.*
> *With our thoughts we make the world."*
> *~ Gautama Buddha ~*

29 DAYS is an interactive series of courses that serve as your very own personal coach. Each course is designed to eliminate an undesirable habit or add a positive one. These courses will change your thoughts, fears, beliefs and attitudes in one area at a time, and it will do it in a way that has never been done before, because it is different from any program ever created. It *does* come with some big promises, but it *doesn't* leave you on your own to figure things out.

---

29 DAYS is designed to generate gentle, effortless, forward momentum – every day.

Throughout this book I have quoted a number of authors who have had a profound impact on my life and this philosophy. People like Zig Ziglar, Robert Maurer, Ph.D., Dr. Maxwell Maltz, Earl Nightingale, Deepak Chopra M.D. and Robert Ringer are just a few of the giants in the world of self-help and motivational change who have positively impacted countless people.

29 DAYS sprang from two decades of my search for a *reliable* way to eliminate unwanted habits. Over twenty years of reading how-to material, attending seminars, and hiring a personal coach, I was still yearning for a better way to acquire good habits and forever eliminate the bad ones. I have attended a number of seminars that promised life-changing results only to be disappointed in the end because they failed to deliver the long-term success for either myself or the people I interviewed. In fact, most of the people I met at seminars could be classified as "seminar junkies." They would admit to attending four or five "life-changing" seminars a year!

On a personal level, I found the motivational books, videos and audio programs were wonderfully entertaining, informative, and generally helpful. In fact, the sources I referenced throughout this book have had a very positive effect on me. But in spite of that, there was often a missing ingredient when it came to making permanent change for many of the people I met.

So, after years of research, I have found a simple, step-by-step process that will change our behaviors – permanently.

29 DAYS combines a number of philosophies, recent breakthrough discoveries of the human brain and the latest communication technology.

Each course will interact with you, twice each day for twenty-nine days, to positively change one significant area of your life at a time.

INTRODUCTION

Give a man a fish and you feed him for a day.
Teach a man to fish and you feed him for a lifetime.
~ Chinese Proverb

29 DAYS ... to a habit you want! is going to teach you *how* to fish. It has one purpose – to help you to independently make positive and permanent changes in your life.

Experience has taught us that if we want to make changes through willpower then those changes will be temporary at best. We also know that if the process is too difficult, it will seldom be followed. We further know that if we try to change too much too quickly, our *self-image* will never buy into it, which will result in nothing but frustration. And finally, a lot of detailed instructions that leave us completely on our own will also lead to a high rate of failure. There are certain principles and formulas to follow that will create the foundation for success and permanent results.

Many how-to programs have a lot of suggestions on how to muster willpower, set goals and repeat affirmations, and they will often work ... temporarily. They're much like diets. All diets will work if we can follow the instructions! But when someone goes on a diet, what is their goal? Is it to go on a diet? Is it to lose weight? The answer to both questions would seem to be yes. So if diets *always work* why do they have such a bad reputation? Studies show that 97% of weight-loss programs fail to achieve permanent results! In fact, most people will put on *more weight* following the completion of a diet because a diet is not a lifestyle change, it's a temporary and strenuous procedure. The other problem with diets, and many of the "how-to" programs, is that they focus on the effect (weight, or the unwanted habit) instead of the cause (attitudes, fears, beliefs and self-image). It's the hole-in-the-bucket syndrome. If you have a hole in your bucket and you're trying to keep the bucket full of water, does it make more sense to find ways of continually adding more water to the bucket or would it be wiser to spend time and effort on repairing the bucket?

29 DAYS is not interested in helping you attain short-term results. These courses are designed to show you how to instill permanent change that will be with you for your lifetime. It's a step-by-step process that cannot fail if you really desire to eliminate a bad habit, or to instill a good habit.

In *29 DAYS* we will guide you towards your goal each and every day. We will show you the proper way to create goals, the right way to take minute action steps while prompting you to ask the *right questions* that will draw available forces to you. All your habits have been programmed whether you are aware of it or not. The good news is that since you were able to install habits you didn't like, you're also able to install habits you desire.

To be successful at any undertaking, any undertaking at all, requires a certain set of rules that must be followed. No exceptions. These rules are the following:

- ✓ **You must have a specific goal.**
- ✓ **It has to be believable to you (self-image) or it will never see completion**
- ✓ **There must be a specific plan to attain that goal.**
- ✓ **There must be a specific and systematic schedule to attain your goal.**
- ✓ **You must have the people and/or the support to help you achieve your desired outcome.**

The 29 DAY courses incorporate all of the above.

You may wish to change a variety of things about yourself, and *29 DAYS* will continually broaden its scope to address many changes that you may desire. We will design courses such as: "*29 DAYS ... to Forgiveness*" or "*29 DAYS ... to a Lifetime of Exercise*." For simplicity's sake throughout this book we will use weight loss for our examples of permanent change.

> Note: The same five rules listed above
> apply to any desirable change.

How Does It Work?

The courses are divided into four weeks with each week having a specific purpose. The four weeks are broken down as:

1. **Commitment and Awareness,**
2. **Preparation for Action,**
3. **Taking Action and**
4. **Staying the Course or, to put it another way, Permanent Lifestyle.**

Within these four weeks are the five steps necessary to attain any goal:

— Step One

Each course has a specific goal in mind. (Quit Smoking, Save Money etc.)

— Step Two

We will guide you toward the correct way to set your goal. Through this procedure you will lay down new mental (neuron) tracks that will harness untapped forces and build unshakable self-confidence. (This concept will be explained in detail later in the book.)

— Step Three

We will be in contact with you at least twice each day (via email) as we walk with you step-by-step toward achieving your goal. We do this through examples, stories, encouragement, prompting questions and generally changing the way you think about this goal or challenge. (This step is a scientifically proven process that will be discussed later in the book.)

— Step Four

Each day you will be required to take a very simple step that will guide you toward completing your goal. This step may be as simple as writing your goal in your journal, reading something we send to you, noticing your tendencies and recurring thoughts, visualizing your goal for a few moments, or simply responding to us by email, which will indicate to your virtual coach that you have reviewed the information for the day.

— Step Five

You and your program will combine forces to become "your daily coach." This unbeatable combination will help you to maintain your focus and commitment. All these steps are purposely designed to enlist the support of the most powerful force in the universe, as well as the one that's closest to home, your subconscious mind. With the blessing and support of your subconscious mind you can achieve anything that you can conceive.

29 DAYS is based on immutable scientific laws and a carefully structured process. Each day you will be guided and inspired toward achieving your specific goal through awareness and a gradual change in the way you think about this particular area of your life. You will quickly see that your mind, seemingly of its own volition, will be reviewing your goal over and over. By about day ten you will catch yourself thinking about your goal even when you weren't consciously focusing on it.

What is the key to real change? Instilling a new habit. Goals you thought were too difficult will be systematically broken down (by this course and your inner-thought process) into easy-to-follow steps so that in a surprisingly short period of time, you will have achieved your seemingly impossible goal. In keeping with the Chinese proverb of "How to Fish," *29 DAYS* will give you the know-how and the confidence to successfully "catch fish" or in this case – change the things you wish to change – and more importantly keep them changed all the days of your life.

So here's our promise: Using the *29 DAYS* courses and selecting the program that aligns with your desired change, you will successfully change that area about yourself, quickly, effortlessly and permanently!

— <u>PART ONE</u> —

Understanding the
Challenges to Change

CHAPTER ONE
What Is a Habit?

Before we dive into the philosophy and workings of *29 DAYS*, it's important to define our definition of *habit*.

People will often argue endlessly about something only to find that they were either arguing the same point or worse, two totally different issues. Suppose one day you and I were discussing former U.S. President Bill Clinton, and I asked you this simple question; "Do you think Bill Clinton is an honest guy?" In reality your answer doesn't mean anything until you and I agree on our definition of honest. What might be considered honest to you might be considered grand larceny to me. Neither you, nor I, may be right in our interpretation of *honest*, but that's not necessary for us to have a meaningful discussion on this topic. What's crucial to our discussion is that we both agree on the definition of honest. Anything other than that is simply a case of you talking, and me waiting, and then me talking and you waiting. Without an understanding of the main point – in this instance our definition of honest, then rational discussion and communication is impossible.

So, with that being said, what is a *habit?*

> A habit is a recurrent, often unconscious pattern of behavior that is acquired through frequent repetition.

Yikes! Can we get that any drier?! Okay, that's a dictionary definition. To add to that, our definition of habits are those things we do that seem to happen almost of their own volition: like overeating, being negative, chain smoking or procrastinating. Have you ever described someone as being "habitually" late? But habits aren't limited to negative things. Many of our habits are desirable. How about a habit of always being complimentary, or looking for the positive in situations? How about the habit of being punctual?

> Habits are things that we do with very little conscious effort.

How are new habits formed?

New habits are formed by thinking new thoughts and forming new pathways in the brain. Therefore, the more you think a particular thought and/or perform a particular action, the quicker you build up the pathway and create the muscle memory to support it.

> *"Our self-image and our habits tend to go together. Change one and you will automatically change the other. The word 'habit' originally meant a garment or clothing... Our habits are literally garments worn by our personalities. They are not accidental, or happenstance. We have them because they fit us. They are consistent with our self-image and our entire personality pattern. When we consciously and deliberately develop new and better habits, our self-image tends to outgrow the old habits and grow into the new pattern."*
> *~ Dr. Maxwell Maltz - Psycho-Cybernetics*

CHAPTER TWO
The Philosophy of Permanent Change

In order for you to enjoy permanent change, you're going to alter the way you think – at least about one particular goal – because if you don't change how you think, you won't change.

> *The world we have created is a product of our thinking;*
> *it cannot be changed without changing our thinking.*
> *~ Albert Einstein*

It doesn't matter if your goal is to lose weight, quit smoking, start an exercise program, stop being negative – or (start being positive), learn to save money or learn to be punctual, every desire for change is within your effortless grasp.

I suspect you're thinking "Ya, right! I've heard this before. What's the catch?"

There's no catch. You simply must *want to change* and if you really want to change, I can absolutely promise success, and the input on your part is going to be minimal. In fact it may seem almost effortless.

It is a proven fact that our thoughts shape our world. Our beliefs affect the way we perceive the world and our beliefs always precede our behavior to reinforce our perception. In effect, our world is not so much experienced by what happens to us, but rather how we *interpret* and *react* to what happens to us. We've all seen children fall down and skin their knees, and we've also witnessed two drastically different responses to a skinned knee. One child will cry and scream and carry on as if he's just been put through the Medieval Inquisition, and another child will merely wince, wipe the blood and tears away and continue to play as if nothing happened. Same experience, two drastically different reactions.

So why would two children react so differently to the same experience? One child thought skinning his knee was a major catastrophe; the other child thought it was just a scrape. If you change how you think, then change will become effortless and permanent. What you think about becomes your truth. How you view yourself becomes your reality. Every thought you think helps to form your future.

In his book, *Creating Health*, Deepak Chopra writes:

> *… for any diet* to be permanently successful, you have to enjoy being on it. In fact you should not feel like you're on a diet at all. Everyone should eat a weight-controlling and healthful diet, not because he thinks it is good for him and will make him lose weight, but because he would honestly prefer not to eat anything else.*
>
> * You may substitute the word "change" or "habit" for diet.

Acquiring habits that are born of a change of attitude and thought, as opposed to willpower, is our goal.

(In the introduction we said that throughout PART ONE, we would use "losing weight" as our recurring example, but bear in mind that the "29 DAYS template" will work for any change you desire.)

If you think losing weight is going to be painful, difficult, and impossible, then it will be. If, on the other hand, you think that losing weight will be painless and inspiring, then that's what it will be. In other words it's not the experience itself, it's your attitude or view *of* the experience. If you have even the slightest doubt about this statement, all you have to do is look at the current fad of "piercing" that is popular within a segment of our society. To the vast majority being stabbed with a metal prong in the imaginative places that piercing is done, would be considered, at the very least, border-line torture. But that being said, for those folks wearing the jewelry in those imaginative body cavities, it's an experience that brings pride and pleasure. It's all in how you view a thing.

This course will ensure that you view the experience in a pleasurable way. In fact we are going to ensure that it will be so painless, and the steps so manageable, that you may want to move faster than we suggest.

22 ~ 29 DAYS ... to a habit you want!

As you will see, our method is to give you first-hand experience, but at the same time we will work with you, guide you, prompt you and encourage you. While you are gaining the experience and learning how to change your habitual thinking, we're right there with you while you learn the fundamental steps of helping yourself. When you know how to help yourself, you can achieve any goal you desire.

Some Guarantees Deliver Everything They Promise … but Ultimately Nothing!

I'll always remember the story my father told me about a so-called guaranteed solution to eliminate the hated potato beetle. My father was raised on an agricultural farm during the late 30s and early 40s. They had a large variety of crops, which included an assortment of fruits and vegetables. A nice selection of crops inevitably attracts the usual suspects. In this case it was the hated and feared potato beetle. If you thought that the third and fourth plagues of gnats and flies that Moses, Pharaoh and the Egyptians suffered through were horrific, that was a mere nuisance compared to the voracious potato beetle! A farmer could go to bed at dusk with a perfectly healthy crop and wake up to see his field stripped of leaves before breakfast. What makes the potato beetle so devastating is its proliferation and unmatched ability to develop resistance to virtually every chemical that's been used against it.

The local fruit and vegetable distributor was the life-blood of the community, for it was here that the neighboring farmers would gather to purchase fertilizer, seed, and the necessary range of equipment from ladders to tractors. It was the perfect place to trade stories, tell hard luck tales, gossip and to discuss methods of combating the potato scourge. As the suggestions, laments and woes of impending doom were being lobbed about, one of the farmers noted a small advertisement in the *Farmer's Almanac*. The ad claimed to have documented proof that this solution offered a 100% success rate in killing the pesky potato beetle. The ad said something to the effect that if you mailed $1.15 in either cash or a teller's check to *The Beetle Bug Solution* at the address listed below, you would be given the "secret weapon" that killed this scourge every time and without fail. It guaranteed that no potato beetle has ever, or could ever, survive this ingenious weapon. It was further promised that the solution would be mailed the very day your money arrived and of course this assurance was backed with an iron-clad money-back guarantee.

Well, there was immediate skepticism to such a claim, but as these things are prone to do, the offer proved irresistible. After all, as one farmer pointed out, "What do we have to lose? If it doesn't work we're guaranteed our money back." That line of logic seemed to hold up under the weight of analysis as the farmers went their various ways.

The following day the neighborhood postman collected a satchel full of envelopes addressed to *The Beetle Bug Solution*. Well it wasn't two weeks later that the guaranteed solutions were delivered. When the anxious recipients tore open their packages it was a sight to behold. There in the little brown envelope was the secret weapon. They found two small blocks of wood and the typed instructions for their exact use. The instructions were short, succinct, and elegantly simple to follow. They read:

> To kill the potato beetle, place it on one of the blocks of wood, and before it can escape, smash down hard on it with the other block. It works every time!

As you can imagine, it took some time for the story to come out since no one wanted to admit they had been duped by such an obvious con. But eventually such a beautiful swindle had to be accepted for what it was, and the locals had a good laugh at their own expense. When someone suggested that "Something ought to be done about this kind of larceny," and that "The lying cheat who sold this malarkey should be locked up for a thousand years," an old wag elegantly pointed out, "The ad, the materials and the instructions did exactly as they promised!"

29 DAYS' Guarantees Are Not Slight of Hand or Print
They're based on five key steps.

Let's review the five keys to success that were outlined earlier in this chapter. To be successful at any undertaking, any undertaking at all, a certain set of rules must be followed. No exceptions. These steps are the following:

1. **You must have a specific goal.**
2. **You must find it believable or it will never see completion.**
3. **You must have a specific plan to attain your goal.**
4. **You must have a specific and systematic schedule to attain your goal.**
5. **You must have the people and/or the support to help you achieve your desired outcome.**

29 DAYS will teach you the simple techniques towards creating permanent change and lasting results. Once you've developed the "self-confidence" and "know how", you will be able to initiate change in every area of your life using the exact same formula. The only kind of change we want, the only kind of change that is really worthwhile, is the change that will have you walking to the river's edge with the confidence that you can catch a fish whenever you desire. In other words instilling the confidence and the knowledge to make changes in your life that will literally stay with you *for* the rest of your life.

It's important to acknowledge the fact that a deeply entrenched habit has strong emotional bonds. People with a long history of low self-esteem won't transform themselves into highly confident individuals in twenty-eight days, but they can transform one area of their lives in twenty-eight days and thus begin to build the basis of a positive-belief-system and the crucial foundation that will transform them into a self-confident person.

Because our focus in *29 DAYS* is targeted toward specific goals, such as *losing weight, becoming positive, quitting smoking* or *saving money,* etc. you can be assured that you're tackling a manageable goal. Now imagine if you simply changed two or three habits each year. What kind of a person would you become in five years? Needless to say the change would be nothing short of extraordinary!

All of us were heavily programmed when we were too young to think for ourselves. Most of our thoughts about our capabilities, behaviors and what's right and wrong were instilled at a very early age, before we were even aware. You could spend years in counseling to uncover why you're afraid of achieving your goals, or you can simply overwrite the problem by changing your thoughts and beliefs about your capabilities, which is exactly what *29 DAYS* will do.

CHAPTER THREE
The Principles of Success

29 DAYS is based on *two* fundamental principles of success:

Principle of Success #1:

- **Patience and perseverance**
  I bet you're thinking "Oh crap, this sounds hard already!" Stay with me, I know it sounds hard but in this application it really isn't. Although patience and perseverance are two distinct words, in our context they are practically interchangeable. Patience is not passive and should never be confused with idleness, in fact it's quite the contrary: It's active, it's concentrated strength, and it's perseverance. To persevere is to prevail. The basic application of patience and perseverance are crucial to your lasting success – and ironically – they are your quickest and most effortless path to permanent change.

Principle of Success #2:

- **The belief and support from your inner-self, which can also be summed up as simple self-confidence.**
  Every successful undertaking in mankind's history has been built on patience and perseverance, *and* the self-confidence to not only undertake a task, but to continue at precisely the point when both patience and perseverance may be running low, you know, that point when everything seems to be going wrong.

In today's society of instant gratification and instant results, our patience and perseverance toward a new goal may be running low by the third day! That is exactly when *29 DAYS* will help to overcome self-doubt, negativity and impatience.

"A journey of a thousand miles must begin with the first step."
~ Lao Tzu

No truer words were ever spoken, *but* equally important are all the successive steps to complete the journey. *29 DAYS* will walk with you through the entire journey to make sure you fulfill your desire.

The Tortoise and The Hare

Do you remember the famous story of the Tortoise and the Hare? It's chock full of the principles of patience, perseverance and self-confidence.

Once upon a time there was a Hare who, boasting how he could run faster than anyone else, was forever teasing Tortoise for its slowness. Then one day, the irate Tortoise answered back: "Who do you think you are? There's no denying you're fast, but even you can be beaten!" The Hare squealed with laughter.

"Beaten in a race? By whom? Not you, surely! I bet there's nobody in the world that can win against me, I'm so speedy. If you think you or anyone else can beat me, why don't you try?" teased the Hare.

Annoyed by such bragging, the Tortoise accepted the challenge. A course was planned, and the next day at dawn they stood at the starting line. The Hare yawned sleepily as the meek Tortoise trudged slowly off.

When the Hare saw how painfully slow his rival was, he decided, half asleep on his feet, to have a quick nap. "Take your time!" he said. "I'll have forty winks and catch up with you in a minute." The Hare woke with a start from a fitful sleep and gazed round, looking for the Tortoise. But the creature was only a short distance away, having barely covered a third of the course.

Breathing a sigh of relief, the Hare decided he might as well have breakfast too, and off he went to munch some cabbages he had noticed in a nearby field. But the heavy meal and the hot sun made his eyelids droop. With a careless glance at the Tortoise, now halfway along the course, he decided to have another snooze before flashing past the winning post. And smiling at the thought of the look on the Tortoise's face when it saw the Hare speed by, he fell fast asleep and was soon snoring happily. The sun started to sink below the horizon, and the Tortoise, who had been plodding towards the winning post since morning, was scarcely a yard from the finish. At that very point, the Hare woke with a jolt. He could see the Tortoise a speck in the distance and away he dashed. He leapt and bounded at a great rate, his tongue lolling, and gasping for breath. Just a little more and he'd be first at the finish. But the Hare's last leap was just too late, for the Tortoise had beaten him to the winning post. Poor Hare! Tired and in disgrace, he slumped down beside the Tortoise who was silently smiling at him.

"Slowly does it every time!" he said.

There are a lot of life's lessons in this short story!

Let's take a closer look at our humble hero and notice the many qualities of character that allowed him to win.

- As noted, he's humble and he readily acknowledges the good in others:
  "There's no denying you're swift," he says to the Hare.

- He's knowledgeable and confident. He knows that everyone and everything *can* be beaten:
  "Who do you think you are? There's no denying you're swift, but even you can be beaten!"

  The Tortoise knows his history. He knows that it doesn't matter if we're talking about Muhammad Ali defeating the "unbeatable" George Foreman, Buster Douglas defeating the "unbeatable" Mike Tyson, The Duke of Wellington defeating Napoleon, the Allies defeating Nazi Germany, Jonas Salk and Albert Sabin defeating Polio, or ourselves overcoming an addiction or undesirable character trait, every seemingly unbeatable foe can be defeated.

- Our Tortoise hero is "human"; even *he* gets angry:
  "Then one day, the irate Tortoise answered back: Who do you think you are?"

- He willingly accepts a daunting challenge:
  "I bet there's nobody in the world who can win against me, I'm so speedy. Now, why don't you try?" Annoyed by such bragging, the Tortoise accepted the challenge.

- He's patient, determined, purposeful and *not* prone to discouragement or outside influence:
  "The Hare woke with a start from a fitful sleep and gazed round, looking for the Tortoise. But the creature was only a short distance away, having barely covered a third of the course."

- He has focus and staying power – perseverance:
  "The sun started to sink below the horizon, and the Tortoise, who had been plodding towards the winning post since morning, was scarcely a yard from the finish."

- The Tortoise knows how to harvest and enjoy the fruits of his labor:
  "Tired and in disgrace, he slumped down beside the Tortoise who was silently smiling at him. Slowly does it every time!" he said.

Like the Tortoise, when you combine the two fundamental principles (patience and perseverance) together with self-confidence, you will be guaranteed success, and you will find yourself reaching your goals quicker and with less effort than you would have ever thought possible.

If you ever catch yourself thinking that you're the overmatched-underdog, or that life has simply stacked too many obstacles against you, try to remember the story of the humble tortoise. History is abundant with "tortoise tales" of ordinary people winning against seemingly impossible odds.

— <u>PART TWO</u> —

Uncovering and Understanding Our Greatest Foe: FEAR

CHAPTER FOUR
The Unlimited (or Limiting) Power of Your Inner-self and Why We Fail

In all likelihood we don't change what we want to change because on a subconscious level the kind of change we are wishing for appears to be too hard and too painful. Our inner self-image refuses to buy in.

In 1960, Dr. Maxwell Maltz, M.D., a plastic surgeon, wrote the timeless classic, *Psycho-Cybernetics*. After thirty-five years of study and observation, he concluded that a person's actions, feelings, behaviors, and even abilities, are consistent with his or her self-image. In other words, you will become the sort of person you think and see yourself being. In Dr. Maltz's words he wrote:

> *I would argue that the most important psychological discovery of modern times is the discovery of the self-image. By understanding your self-image and by learning to modify it and manage it to suit your purposes, you gain incredible confidence and power.*
>
> *This self-image is our own conception of the "sort of person I am." It has been built up from our own beliefs about ourselves. Most of which have unconsciously been formed from our past experiences, our success and failures, our humiliations, our triumphs, and the way other people have reacted to us, especially in early childhood. From all these we mentally construct a self (or a picture of self). Once an idea or a belief about ourselves goes into this picture it becomes "truth," as far as we personally are concerned. We do not question its validity, but proceed to act upon it 'just as if it were true'.*

The self-image then controls what you can and cannot accomplish, what is difficult or easy for you, even how others respond to you just as certainly and scientifically as a thermostat controls the temperature in your home.

In short, your entire life is a perfect reflection of your self-image. Each of us will act in direct accordance with how we see ourselves. In fact, it's not possible to act otherwise.

As a corollary to that, I will say that willpower is tail-chasing. Creating a desired self-image is tantamount to success.

The *29 DAYS* courses are committed to shining a light into the dark recesses of our inner thoughts that have held us back because of a fragile self-image.

As you're going to find out, positive change won't be difficult because you are going to change the way you think about it. If you found change was difficult in the past it was only because you *thought* it was difficult.

In *Hamlet*, Shakespeare wrote: "*There is nothing either good or bad, but thinking makes it so.*"

So let's rephrase that Shakespearean quote: "If we *think* it so … it *will* be so."

The modern mantra of "no pain no gain" is often associated with a right of passage or badge of honor, somewhat like having your dentist skip the anesthesia when he's drilling for a cavity. It might make for some bragging rights, if you can stand the pain, but what's the point?

29 DAYS is not designed to avoid pain and heartache, because neither "pain" nor "heartache" will ever come into play. In fact, if this course ever *does* become painful, let *that* serve as a warning sign that you're *not* following the course properly. This course is about effortless and lasting change, not fleeting, teeth-clenched, short-term willpower.

How We Often Set Ourselves Up for Certain Failure: "The New Year's Eve Syndrome"

Let's look at a some "typical" examples of people who finally say "That's it, I've got to change!"

The tactic they employ is teeth-clenched, head down, smash-through-the-wall change – a sure recipe for failure.

It's New Year's Eve. "After tonight I'm determined to change my life. I'm going into the New Year with a fresh start and a new attitude. I am certain that *I can* and *will* change. *I will* become a new person!"

Sandy is forty pounds overweight. She hates the way she looks and the thought of getting into a bathing suit and being seen in public causes her to break into a cold sweat. Sandy has always found great comfort in junk food, soda pop and long stretches flopped in front of the TV. But it's New Year's Eve and Sandy has hit the wall. She vows to herself that this is the year for positive change. She's going to join a womans' fitness club, throw out all the junk-food in the house, and buy a couple of "How To" books on getting into shape. She vows to start the New Year with a vengeance.

WHAT'S LIKELY TO HAPPEN: By about day three something will go wrong. Sandy's boss will reprimand her, or she'll imagine that she heard someone call her a "fat cow" or she'll pull a muscle in her new workout regimen, and wham, she'll be back on the couch with the snacks and clicker just as sure as sh--, God made little green apples!

WHAT DID SANDY'S INNER SELF SAY?: "Sandy my dear, I haven't said anything for three days about this diet and exercise stuff only because I was laughing too hard to speak. But now that we've both had a chance to come back to earth let's be serious. *You* join a womans' fitness club, and stop eating junk food? Come on, who are you kidding? Life isn't easy. Hey, relaxing after a long, hard day at work is *your* right. After all, so what if you're a few pounds overweight? People who are the "so-called" perfect weight don't seem any happier. We all have our vices. Life has to have some fun. There's more to living than just work and exercise!"

"Well, if you put it that way", Sandy replies to her inner self, "I suppose you're right. I guess I *was* being unrealistic. I'll get the snacks, you see what's on TV!"

JASON – AGE 28

Jason is a shy little wallflower. He's the kind of guy who goes to the beach and actually *does* get sand kicked in his face. For as long as Jason can remember he's been intimidated by loud, aggressive people. He hates contact sports and most sports in general. Jason's idea of a good night is reading the latest computer programming manuals or playing video games. But it's New Year's Eve and Jason is sitting at home, alone, in his parents' basement. As he sits watching the Times Square celebration on TV, he decides right then and there that he's reached the end of his rope. "No more Mr. Nice guy. If Jack Lalane can transform his life from a ninety-nine pound weakling, then so can I." Jason commits to joining a health club, hiring a personal trainer and getting pumped. At the same time he's going to join a martial arts studio, learn to fight and look like Arnold Schwarzenegger in nine months.

WHAT'S LIKELY TO HAPPEN: Jason might get as far as joining a club, and he may even begin a workout regimen – provided he goes so far as to hire a personal trainer. Jason will be so afraid of letting his trainer down he may actually stay with his workout schedule for a couple of weeks. But at some point between the martial arts classes and the gym workout, Jason is going to look in the mirror and see the same shy, skinny kid who absolutely hates what he's putting himself through. His subconscious will take over and he'll end up pulling a muscle or twisting his ankle and that will be his ticket to flee this madness.

WHAT DID JASON'S INNER SELF SAY? "Hey, whoa, slow down little guy, have you completely lost your mind? You are a square peg and that exercise stuff is a round hole! You are born to do gentle things. *You*, learn to fight?! With a video controller yes, with your fists … forget it. Hey why don't you worry about getting your own apartment? After all, you're twenty-eight years old and you're still living with your parents. You're just not cut out for that macho stuff."

LORA – AGE 33

Lora hates meeting people. Whenever she's introduced to anyone she never knows what to say. As for striking up a conversation with anyone of the opposite sex … forget it. On top of being painfully shy, she thinks her breasts are too small and her nose is too big. Lora is "celebrating" New Year's Eve alone in her apartment. As she thinks about the past thirty-three years of her life she decides it's time for change. Massive change. Starting tomorrow she vows that this is the year she's going to come out of her shell, and meet the man of her dreams. Right then and there she decides she's going to join Toastmasters, buy some sexy new clothes and throw off the shackles of feeling inferior. After all, she is woman … watch her roar!

WHAT'S LIKELY TO HAPPEN: Lora makes the call to Toastmasters and agrees to attend the first meeting as a guest the following evening. Lora spends the next day building mental images of awkward introductions and being forced to make impromptu speeches in front of complete strangers. That night she forces herself to attend the meeting and it's even worse than she had imagined. Everyone she meets asks her to say something about herself. She stammers and stutters and finally excuses herself to go to the washroom. On the way to the ladies' room she passes the coat rack and almost without realizing it she grabs her jacket and bee-lines to the parking lot. "What could I have possibly been thinking?" she asks herself as she's running to her car.

WHAT DID LORA'S INNER SELF SAY? "Lora, we need to get a grip on reality. You like meeting new people about as much as they like meeting you. It's a painful, awkward experience for everyone involved; so why don't you give yourself and everyone else a break and forget the whole thing. For your entire life the only place you've been comfortable is in the background. You're a good person just as you are. The world's got enough out going social misfits. You enjoy your own company so what's wrong with that?" After a nanosecond of thought, Lora agrees and retreats to her life of solitude.

Do any of these scenarios sound familiar? Not that *you* have ever made radical New Year's Eve vows like this … but perhaps you're familiar with some wild resolutions that *other people* have made?

Why didn't Sandy, Jason or Lora have the slightest chance of achieving their resolutions and goals? Because their hopes were one thing and their inner beliefs about their capabilities were something else.

Four basic reasons for their failure:
1. They attempted far more than they were mentally ready for.
2. They expected (wanted) change to happen almost instantaneously without properly preparing for that change.
3. They were acting out of desperation and fear, rather than from conviction, belief and the support from their inner-self.
4. They failed to enlist some form of external support.

---

29 DAYS will guide you to your goals by addressing each of the 4 causes of failure.

Most of us are like that rabbit in the *Tortoise & Hare*, speed is everything! We want results and we want them *now!* In fact, yesterday would be preferable.

Since we know that demanding instantaneous results is *one cause* of almost certain disaster, let's delve further into some *other causes* of failure.

CHAPTER FIVE
Fear and the Futility of Expecting Instant Results

Why Is Change So Difficult?

If we *know* what is good for us (lose weight, save money, be more positive, quit smoking) and we *know* what to do to affect the change (eat less, spend less, look for the good, don't light up) then why, why, why is it so difficult?

In a word, FEAR.

Our minds will seldom accept overnight change. Our brains* are hardwired to resist radical change; in fact as you'll soon see, it's a built-in survival mechanism.

If our minds will not accept instant change then how do we explain people who stop smoking cold turkey, or people who have never previously exercised suddenly begin a lifelong workout program? What about people who suddenly change their diets and eating habits into a permanently healthy lifestyle?

Traditionally these "overnight" changes were either falsely interpreted or they are akin to an epiphany, a transcendence, or a "Saul on the road to Damascus" miracle awakening. Although we're all aware of examples of people's lives being suddenly transformed, such as a crip-

Note: For clarification of terms, the brain is generally considered to be the physical anatomy and the mind is what the brain generates through its activity. Eastern philosophy and New Age thinking tend to suggest this view is backward. To them, it's the mind that is the source of thought, and the brain simply reacts to what the mind feeds it. In 29 Days, we use the words "mind" and "brain" interchangeably because neither concept will interfere with your results.

pling addiction suddenly and effortlessly cast aside, or someone achieving instantaneous spiritual enlightenment, in every case these spectacular events are neither predictable nor controllable.

To say that we're wired to resist change, and that our resistance stems from fear, does not discount the fact that many of us *have* managed to initiate radical changes in our lives – *when* and *if* we've hit the so-called "wall." You know the place, like our examples of Sandy, Jason and Lora, where you suddenly say, "That's it! I've had it! I'm never going to do that again!"

"So," you might reasonably conclude, "there goes your theory of *not* being able to make radical changes at will." Not so.

There's no doubt that radical, and instantaneous change does happen. It happens to people everyday, but is it something we can do on command? Is it something that we can do at will and with other, or all, areas of our lives? Can we sustain it? Can we make it a habit? The overwhelming evidence says no!

Let me give you a personal example of how I managed an "overnight" change.

I took up smoking when I was fourteen and by the age of sixteen I was a "committed" smoker. Within three years I had managed to ratchet my daily intake of cigarettes to two packs per day. By the time I was twenty-one, I was up to three packs per day – which at the time I thought must be close to the physical limits since there are only so many hours in the day, that was until I began waking up during the night to … you guessed it, "enjoy" another cigarette.

Needless to say that over the years I had managed to "quit" a number of times. I often joked how easy it was to quit since I had managed the feat so readily. In reality it wasn't quitting, it was just a temporary suspension, that never lasted more than a few days. I was a bona fide smoker. In fact, I actually couldn't imagine life worth living without cigarettes. After all, if I quit how could I ever again enjoy talking on the telephone without the aid and comfort of a smoke? How could I ever enjoy a beer without an accompanying cigarette? Enjoying a delicious meal and relaxing in front of the TV would have been "empty" without the perfect finishing touch, a cigarette. These smoky pleasures permeated every area of my life, all day long and well into the night. I simply couldn't imagine living without them.

But like every seasoned smoker knows, it's a life sentence to slavery. Like all smokers I always told myself that I would quit before it was too late, whatever that meant. Even though it was less expensive to buy cigarettes by the carton, I never did because I always thought, "What happens if I buy a ten-pack carton and decided to quit with only a part of the carton used up? I mean, what would I do with the other packs? What a waste. In fact, wouldn't I then keep smoking just to finish off the carton?"

Nobody ever accused a smoker's thoughts toward the addiction as rational!

As a smoker I loathed this part of my life. I was angry and disgusted that I was so controlled by my dependancy on what was such an utterly destructive habit. Then one day I decided that I would quit, but I also decided that I was definitely *not* going to try to quit *that* day. Instead I decided to take a deep look at the psychological bondage that I had tied myself to. Instead of trying to cut back, or quit, I actually forced myself to increase my daily intake.

Now remember this was many years ago, when smokers weren't looked on as the pariahs they are today. Back then you could smoke on airplanes, public transportation; aside from smoking in church, you could smoke anywhere you pleased and nobody gave it a second thought. So when I say I was going to increase my daily intake, I literally began to light one cigarette from the previous. Were there many times that I had just finished a cigarette and didn't feel like smoking another at that moment? Almost always. But I forced myself to smoke it anyway because if cigarettes are so pleasurable, why would I possibly deprive myself of *all* the pleasure I could garner?

With each cigarette I smoked I really thought about how much I hated it. I was "subconsciously" reprogramming my beliefs that smoking was "pleasurable" and "impossible to quit." This self-imposed torture of continually smoking went on for a couple of weeks, and as you can well imagine, it was beginning to seriously effect my immediate health. I was constantly fatigued and felt unwell. I knew that I was going to quit, I knew that I *had* to quit, but I let the entire fiasco run its course. I knew a change was going to happen, but I really didn't know how or when.

Then came the day. I can recall it as clear as if it happened yesterday. I was twenty-seven years old. I awoke one morning and it quite literally felt like someone was standing on my chest. It was a clear and unmistakable sign. The not-too subtle warning was accompanied by that deep knowing. It was one of those life-defining moments. Either I quit smoking or I would never see forty.

The knowing was so complete that when I got out of bed and looked at my pack of cigarettes I calmly threw them in the garbage, got dressed and went to work. I haven't smoked a cigarette in twenty-three years. Were there times in the ensuing weeks and months that I longed for a cigarette? Occasionally. In fact, years later I might be talking on the phone and the thought of "enjoying" a "pleasant cigarette" would pop into my mind, but the thought was fleeting and carried little substance. My freedom meant far more to me than anything else. To this day, I will still say that my greatest accomplishment was ridding myself of that vile, filthy, disgusting habit. For a long time I thought that I had broken my smoking slavery through willpower. Today I know that nothing could be further from the truth. What I had done was systematically change my thought process. I had slowly but surely began to see my habit and addiction for what it was. When I thought cigarettes were my friends I was completely under their control. When I changed my thinking to realize they were my biggest enemy *I* finally had control. It was then, and only then that I could stop smoking ... permanently!

Now, to underscore my point, even though I used to think that I had quit cold turkey, that's not really the case. Everyone who quits at some point has had their last cigarette. We might think that at that point, they had to quit, cold turkey. Technically this is true, but in reality there was a thought process that had to lead up to that point. In my case there was a particular moment when I said "That's it, I've had it!" but in order to get to that place where I could leave it behind, I had to spend a couple of weeks changing my deepest beliefs about smoking.

When people seem to change deep habits and addictions, 'overnight,' seemingly through the use of willpower, if you were to look closer you will likely find that there was much more involved than what appears on the surface. There are always exceptions but in all likelihood they're too rare to bother with. In fact, *if* one can manage such major change through the use of willpower, then by rights they should be able to transform themselves into a perfect walking, talking, performing human being over night. The sad reality is that change through the instantaneous process of willpower has always produced dismal results.

The instantaneous attempts that are most common are fad diets, austerity vows to eliminate debt, cold turkey, spur of the moment, attempts at quitting smoking or drinking or gambling or the assumption of a new personality by joining a social community.

There are always a few well-publicized success stories that fuel the belief that overnight change is possible and commonplace. These publicized stories often lead us to believe that if we can't initiate the instantaneous change we want, then we must be deficient in personal force or willpower. Nothing could be further from the truth!

> Your willpower will never be stronger than your subconscious mind, no matter what.

Mr. A – The Classic Overachieving Willpower Guy

Most of us know the classic Type A personality. The person who tries to run his life on the fuel of willpower. Type A people are aggressive, impatient, tense and hard driving. They are forever trying to beat a deadline, and relaxing is a foreign concept.

We may all know a Type A who by sheer will manages to quit a debilitating addiction, train for a triathlon, or perform some other life challenging task. This Herculian effort often produces eye-popping results, and it's even quite likely that many of us can think of examples in our *own* lives where we have achieved a goal through determination and massive overnight change. This kind of personal power can be a real confidence builder and an internal source of pride, but it's also very unreliable and can have some devastating effect on our confidence and self-esteem *if*, and inevitably in some area we will, fail.

If personal power was a sure formula for success, then it stands to reason that anyone who ever achieved success through personal power (stop a bad habit or start a good one) should simply be able to duplicate the same formula in every area of his or her life. By this reasoning, within a year or so, our "personal-power-individual" should (in his eyes at least) be totally pleased with every area of his life. As we've all witnessed, this formula may work on occasion, but for broad, long term, meaningful change, it's simply not reliable and will ultimately stack one more failed attempt onto a growing heap. In fact, successive failures can often lead to the debilitating attitude of, "Why bother? I never succeed at anything anyway."

If you happen to be an Type A personality, and you really can achieve your goals through sheer force of will, then good for you.

In the *29 DAYS* courses, our aim is to achieve our goals. *That, and only that,* is our measure of success. If we want to get from the country to the city our goal then is to arrive in the city. It doesn't much matter (to our ultimate goal) if we ride in a Chevy, a Rolls Royce or a bicycle for that matter, the aim is to get to the city. Our arrival – by whatever means - is proof of our success.

Getting back to our Mr. 'A', and his formula for success. We know him to be rather predictable, you know the kind … "I want everything yesterday, and I will get it *all*, even if I have to run through a wall or turn the world upside down to get it!"

For convenience sake, let's call our Type A personality "Arnold", and one day Arnold decides he's going to soften his aggressive personality.

Arnold's day isn't atypical. It is just another one of those days filled with tension and stress. But then late in the afternoon, after chewing out another employee, something happens to "lovable" Arnold. He has a quiet moment and he suddenly realizes that his demeanor and general behavior might actually benefit from some modifications and adjustments. As a result, he decides to try to mellow-out and soften his edges. Just like that!

Arnold realizes that being a bull in a china shop has its limitations and as a result, he decides he wants to modify his behavior for a better relationship with his family, friends and associates. As a result, he decides that starting the very next morning he will begin to enjoy a quiet moment, stop to notice the beauty of his surroundings, offer an uncharacteristic word of encouragement to his employees and take time out to reflect on life. All this will begin the following morning, through sheer force of will.

If you're imagining a Type A person right now, you're probably laughing at the notion. We simply KNOW that that type of behavior is completely foreign to a Type A personality and such radical, overnight behavioral change is highly unlikely.

If Arnold sincerely desires to be a more compassionate soul who takes time for simple moments and sincere communication, he *can* achieve his goal, but he must go about it in the right way. The cold-turkey, willpower approach will fail every single time and it will fail because Arnold will *never* sneak this one past his inner-self!

CHAPTER SIX
Simple Steps Will Sow the Seeds of Belief and Success

Arnold will fail in his attempt because his approach will never be accepted by his inner-self or subconscious mind. His inner-self will laugh hysterically at the very notion. Without the acceptance of his inner-self, any attempt at changing his "core" personality won't last.

For Arnold to make a sustainable personality change, he must take certain steps that will change his core beliefs.

These steps are fundamental to your success. They will work for any person, any personality and in any situation. They will work every time, and they will never fail provided the following conditions are met:

1. **You must sincerely want to change**
2. **You must be willing to change ... gradually (The Way of the Tortoise)**
3. **You must generate gentle, effortless, forward momentum every day ... for twenty-nine days — this will establish the strong foundation for a new lifestyle, and a new way of living.**

John Wooden, one of the most successful college basketball coaches of all time, beautifully phrased this process when he said:

> *"When you improve a little each day, eventually big things occur. When you improve conditioning a little each day, eventually you have a big improvement in conditioning. Not tomorrow, not the next day, but eventually a big gain is made. Don't look for the big, quick improvement. Seek the small improvement one day at a time. That's the only way it happens – and when it happens, it lasts."*

Change Is Difficult because We Instinctively Fear Change

Man is a creature that craves familiarity, and as a result, we form habits and routines (some good and some not so good) that eventually feel comfortable. Have you ever noticed when you sit down to watch television you and your spouse always sit in the same place regardless of who gets there first? Do you have "your" side of the bed? Do you take the same route to the local grocery store or to work even though there might be alternatives that are just as easy or as close? Do you notice when a group of employees gather for regular meetings that within a short period of time everyone has their spot for successive meetings?

The old expression "better the devil you know than the devil you don't" holds true. Taken to an even greater extreme, how often have we read of mistreated children defending their parents? How about spouses finding excuses to stay in abusive marriages or people staying in jobs that they absolutely hate year after year? Even long-term prisoners who have yearned for freedom experience tremendous anxiety as their release date approaches. They've become so accustomed to their prison routine they experience genuine fear of change.

All changes, even positive ones, are scary. Attempts to reach goals through radical or revolutionary action will almost always fail because they heighten fear and cut off the cooperation of our subconscious mind.

The Keys to Goal Achievement

1. Focus or purpose: If you don't have a goal the odds are one-hundred percent that you will not achieve it. 29 DAYS starts you off with an achievable goal and together we make sure it is gentle, measurable, and that you maintain forward momentum. This kind of progress builds unshakeable self-confidence.

2. Sincerity: You must want to achieve it. Don't confuse this with teeth gritted, iron will determination; in fact, it may be quite the contrary. At times you will want to move quicker than 29 DAYS will suggest! But you mustn't force the matter. It's imperative to stay with the system.

3. Slow, consistent, forward momentum: Completely disarms the brain's fear response which will stimulate your inner-self, or subconscious mind, that bottomless well of all possibilities given to each of us at birth.

4. Self-monitoring system: 29 DAYS will guide you each day through interaction and a measurement process as you literally begin to build your picture of progress and ultimate success.

5. Accountability: 29 DAYS will ask you to participate every day whether that's something as basic as sixty seconds of meditation or spending several minutes reading the daily message, or simply acknowledging that it's your "reward" day.

6. Reward Yourself: That's right! 29 DAYS recognizes your participation and progress and the importance that you should also recognize and appreciate your success. This is key to building that unshakeable self-confidence that is the foundation of all success.

Too many people keep their nose so stuck to the grindstone that they wear themselves out even while they're making progress. They make themselves feel like failures even while they're successful. 29 DAYS will be sure that you reward yourself for your steady progress and small, but life-changing, victories.

— <u>PART THREE</u> —

Our Thoughts: The Source of All Good and Bad!

CHAPTER SEVEN
How Gentle Progress Bypasses Our "Hardwired" Brains

Examining Our Incredible Brain

When it comes to character traits and habits, it doesn't really matter whether we say our brain is hardwired from birth or we say to ourselves, "That's just the way I am" or "That trait runs in my family" it still comes down to the same thing – we are the result of programming – genetically, acquired or self-induced. Anyway we look at it, this ingrained programming can and must be bypassed.

Whether we're trying to remove a negative habit or make a positive change, the part that always trips us up, and the prime cause of our failure to make permanent changes in our lives, is that change activates fear. If we want to change, we must bypass fear.

Fear of change is part of being human. The kind of change that causes fear does not have to be catastrophic change to induce it. Fear can be caused by something as simple as ordering a brand new dish at our favorite restaurant (or NOT ordering that dish for the same reason) or taking an unfamiliar route to work.

> The key point is that
> CHANGE CAUSES FEAR
> and
> FEAR CAUSES RESISTANCE.

Fear of change is rooted in the brain's physiology, and when fear takes hold, it can prevent creativity, change and success. To understand this basic law of human nature, its causes and effects, we need to take a quick look at the source – our extraordinary brain.

Without our highly developed brain, mankind would have been lucky to survive a week in the harsh environment of planet earth. Because of our unmatched ability to think and to reason, man rules the earth, but without our brain we are completely defenseless. We cannot swim like the creatures of the sea, we cannot fly like birds, we cannot stand extreme temperatures like the polar bear, lizard or camel, we have no natural camouflage, we are relatively weak against a mammal like the gorilla or lion, and our ground speed is slower than almost all of our natural land predators. In short we cannot outrun, out-swim, hide from or overpower our natural predators, and without our brains man's the most defenseless creature on the planet.

Every psychological theory recognizes that we are made up of several different selves. Our brain has evolved over millions of years leaving us with distinct parts, each with its own function. To further complicate matters we have to coordinate our distinct brains along with two evolving minds: conscious and subconscious. That's a lot of orchestrating!

The Triune Brain

The "Triune Model" or three-part brain theory was developed by Dr. Paul MacLean, Chief of the Laboratory of Brain Research and behavior, National Institute of Mental Health.

The Triune model is based on three stages of brain evolution, the "Reptilian," the "Mammalian" and "Cortex." It is also commonly referred to as the R-complex, the limbic system, and the neocortex. Each of these stages represents a brain evolving over eons of time to the changing circumstances of its environment.

Each brain has its own function and each brain has a "natural tendency" to act in an isolated manner, behaving independently of the other two. Each have their own special intelligence, subjectivity, sense of time, space and memory.

How our three brains work and function

Understanding the basics of how our brains function, and how they relate to our current beliefs, and the way we interpret information can help us understand the process of eliminating negative habits or installing new positive habits. So with that in mind, let's take a quick look at the most extraordinary tools ever created – our brains.

REPTILIAN BRAIN

The reptilian brain may be as much as 300 to 500 million years old. Since it stopped evolving about 200 million years ago, this portion of our brain is essentially the same as in all reptiles. It is involuntary, impulsive and compulsive; it contains programmed responses that are devoted to self-preservation. This part of the brain does not learn from experience. It repeats its programmed behavior over and over. Its function is to watch for enemies and search for prey. Also, the same brain warns us of an approaching car or possible danger in a dark alley.

This brain evolved for survival. It controls basic life functions such as heart rate, reproduction, fighting, fleeing, feeding and breathing. It can be thought of as a life of easy choices: "Can I eat it?" "Should I ignore it?" "Should I run away?"

MAMMALIAN BRAIN

This brain evolved about 100 million years ago. We share this brain with all mammals similar to the way we share our reptilian portion with all reptiles.

For our purposes, we will combine the Reptilian Brain and the Mammalian Brain (the two oldest parts) and call it the subconscious mind.

The mammalian brain contains feelings and emotions. It is playful and the source of maternal care. Mammals will generally tend to their young whereas reptiles usually do not. The mammalian part of the brain provides us with feelings of what is real, true and important. It is the source of our emotions, family and social ties as well as feelings of responsibility, ethics and duty to others.

The mammalian brain, however, is inarticulate in communicating these feelings to the conscious mind. Important features are that the subconscious mind is the source of feelings and it derives its value system by combining both experience and its emotional impact.

THE CORTEX

The cortex represents the third stage of development, and it's what makes humans superior to all other creatures on our planet. This is the creative brain that is responsible for art, science, music, advanced communication, future planning and reason.

The cortex is the conscious part of the mind. An important feature of the conscious brain/mind is that it does not begin to develop until about age three and is not fully developed until about twenty years of age. This late development is why we have so many negative and counterproductive programs in our subconscious minds.

When the emotional part of our brains (subconscious) developed in our early years, we lacked the ability to filter out negative comments from parents, teachers, siblings and friends as well as the ability to select positive programs that would enhance our self-esteem. To compound the problem, we were not then, and even now, aware of most of these programs since we have no memory of them.

In contrast to the subconscious mind, which evolves its value system through emotions, the conscious mind evolves its value system through "rational" interpretation of experience.

The cortex (the conscious mind) will analyze problems and come up with rational solutions, often without the vaguest idea of what is taking place in the old brain, or subconscious mind, which is governed by non-rational feeling.

The old brain *can* bypass the thinking brain's control systems and act out of intense emotions that have been bottled up in the subconscious since childhood. The new brain (cortex), operating in present time, realizes that the person has strength, competence, and self-worth, yet the subconscious continues to trigger ineffective, inappropriate responses to life's challenges based on long-ago programming.

Let's evaluate your understanding of the three brains with this little test. See if you can connect which brain would be responsible for each answer.

1. You're sitting on the beach after a day of sunning and you're hungry. At that moment, what appears to be food, drops down in front of you.
   a. This looks great, and smells great. This might just be my lucky day. _____
   b. Chomp, chomp, gulp. _____
   c. Is it really true? Is this really edible food? _____
2. You're at home eating dinner and the phone rings. The caller says; "If you give me $1,000 I can turn it into a million dollars in less than six months"!
   a. If that's true, why are you wasting your time making these humiliating cold calls?
   _____
   b. Come over, I want to eat you. _____
   c. Sounds great. I'll get the money first thing in the morning.
   _____

3. A self-made billionaire, looking for investors, has a great idea for a new business venture.
    a. This sounds like a no-brainer. This guy has a great idea and he's rich.

    _____

    b. Forget the businessman and his past history. Explain the idea in detail. _____
    c. When can I eat this guy? _____
4. A politician running for office promises a "chicken in every pot and a car in every garage."
    a. Promises, promises. Let's talk reality. _____
    b. This sounds fantastic. You've got my vote. _____
    c. I'll eat both the chicken and the car. Can I eat the politician as well? _____

Let's see how you did.

1. a. mammalian
    b. reptilian
    c. cortex
2. a. cortex
    b. reptilian
    c. mammalian

3. a. mammalian
    b. cortex
    c. reptilian
4   a. cortex
    b. mammalian
    c. reptilian

With this simple picture of our three brains in mind, imagine them as three horses pulling a chariot. If we can get all three brains working in unison toward a common goal, our chariot will move quickly and efficiently to our directed destination. If, on the other hand, each horse is going in its own direction, our chariot will experience a great pull of force, but very little forward or positive direction.

This brings us back to our habits and goals and why positive change is often so difficult.

Fight or Flight? Ah, that Is the Question!

According to our two most primitive brains, everything is either agreeable or disagreeable. Survival is based upon the avoidance of pain (disagreeable) and the recurrence of pleasure (agreeable).

You're planning a winter vacation in the Caribbean so you and your cortex decide that you're going to go on a diet so you'll look your best in a bathing suit. That night however, you and your primitive brains decide to eat a large bag of potato chips.

You attend a how-to seminar and again, you and your cortex decide that you're going to make some serious changes toward enhancing your life. You're going to take up exercise, join a yoga class and take some night courses to increase your skills. Within a few days your primitive brain, or your inner-self, begin to send signals that any form of change is absolutely unacceptable! Soon the idea is all but forgotten.

Why do we self sabotage what we know is best for us?

There are two schools of thought on the culprit. One school of thought blames our self-sabotage on the ... amygdala (a-MIG-duh-luh).

The amygdala, an almond sized and shaped structure located in the mid-brain, can take full credit for man's survival as a species because it controls the fight-or-flight response. Its purpose is to alert the body for action in the case of perceived danger, but in today's world our amygdala is often nothing but a stick in the spokes of our modern lives.

The moment the amygdala detects even the slightest danger it seizes control. Earlier we said that man is a creature that craves familiarity and as a result, we form habits and routines that eventually feel safe and comfortable.

Even things that pose a serious threat to our wellbeing such as overeating, smoking or excessive drinking will not raise an alarm once they're habitual because it doesn't register an internal alarm.

This is a very important concept to grasp!

The amygdala always has its foot resting on the "gas pedal" and it won't hesitate to punch it down at the slightest hint of imminent danger. When the pedal gets pushed, "fight or flight" takes full priority, and all unnecessary functions such as digestion, thought processes and sexual desire are immediately shut down. As you can imagine, for many thousands of years, this automatic reaction to danger has allowed the survival of our species. If we were being stalked by a predator we were obviously in imminent danger. We wouldn't want our brain to stop and consider the percentages of survival, or consider alternate methods while evaluating the situation. We need to survive the next few minutes so that we can live another day to ponder how we can prevent a similar occurrence in the future.

The fight-or-flight response is still crucial today, but it hasn't fully adapted to our rapidly changing world. Although it's not *as* necessary in our modern world we still need the amygdala to safely cross a busy street, flee from a mugger, escape a burning building, overpower an intruder, or rise to some other life-threatening circumstance.

The glitch with the amygdala in today's world is that it's still ready to punch down the physical gas pedal of fight-or-flight even when we wish it would just stay asleep. The amygdala's goal is to make our lives predictable, because change could cause discomfort and anxiety, and change may invite unknown hazards.

Our amygdala can be aroused at even the slightest departure from our regular routines. Our mammalian brain wakens the amygdala at the faintest hint of fear, but that fear can be meeting new people, making a speech, starting a savings program, going to a job interview or starting a new exercise routine.

When alarmed, our amygdala stops other functions such as rational and creative thinking — thoughts that could interfere with our physical ability to run or fight. In fact, any time we attempt to make a departure from our usual safe routines, the amygdala alerts parts of the body to prepare for action — and our access to the cortex, the rational thinking part of the brain, is either restricted or shut down. In fact, it will even go so far as to send messages to you through such means as back pain, fatigue, minor accidents and mental confusion.

If you have the slightest doubt about this, consider the typical reaction we encounter when we're about to take a driver's test, give a speech, write an exam or tee-up a golf ball in front of a crowded club house.

Why would these situations cause our heart rate to increase, our palms to sweat, and our muscles to tense? It's our amygdala sensing fear, which starts up our fight-or-flight survival mechanisms even though it's the very last thing we need at that moment in time.

Fear restricts access to the cortex, which in turn can often result in failure. If we can bypass fear, we can access our cortex and usually enjoy success. Unfortunately the neural connections from the cortex down to the amygdala are less well developed than are connections from the amygdala back up to the cortex. Thus, the amygdala exerts a greater influence on the cortex than vice versa. Once an emotion has been turned on, it is difficult for the cortex to turn it off.

There is practically no limit to the imagined lions and tigers that constantly stalk us; only today they are paper lions and tigers disguised as losing weight, getting a new job, asking someone we admire on a date or meeting a sales goal.

There is a second school of thought that doesn't necessarily point any self-sabotaging fingers at the amygdala, but rather to an *inner child* or *rebellious side* that each of us carries around with us.

Dr. Eric Berne, author of *Games People Play* and creator of *Transactional Analysis*, along with other people in that field, talked about our "child," "adult" and "parent tapes" that are like three voices within us. One is the desirous child; one is the adult who is rational, intelligent, and educated; and one is the parent who tends to be punitive and moralistic.

The inner child is generally a spoiled, inconsiderate personality who demands everything immediately with no regard for cost. This child will violently rebel at the slightest hint of structure. This child is certain that any form of self-discipline will mean becoming a slave to routine, and a complete loss of freedom and fun. We can refer to this rebellious child as our inner demons or as discussed much earlier, our self-image. We all have inner demons. All of us have battled them. We also have the battle scars to prove their existence, those times when we do inexplicably dumb things and cannot say why any rational human being would have acted in that manner.

At any rate, it doesn't much matter whether we are blaming the amygdala, our inner demons, early life self-programming or our flawed self-image, it amounts to the same thing, we have inner challenges that must be overruled.

So what's the solution?

29 DAYS courses are designed to generate gentle, effortless, forward momentum – every day, while being careful not to arouse the amygdala or those inner demons. These small gentle steps engage the cortex, the rational thinking brain, while simultaneously laying down a new roadway for our subconscious thoughts. This new roadway is the superhighway that builds new habits and lasting results.

CHAPTER EIGHT
How Small Actions and Gentle Repetition of Thought Can Transform Our Lives

It's highly likely that you are familiar with the term, "Use it or lose it!" when people are referring to using ones muscles. But this statement is now accepted as fact when referring to our brains as well.

In December 1997, scientist Fred H. Gave, Ph.D. and his colleagues discovered a phenomenon called brain plasticity or neurogenesis. Their discovery revealed that when you stimulate your brain, no matter what your age, your brain will grow new connections that appear as tiny, thin strands — as intricate as a spider web — called DSPs (Dendrite Spine Protuberances). DSPs greatly increase the total number of connections in your brain along with your brain's capacity for achievement!

The term "plasticity" means adaptable, shapeable, changeable and capable of growth and transformation. For many years, scientists believed that we were each born with "hard wiring" in our brains, and that for the rest of our lives we were stuck with, and limited to, what we were given at birth. As it turns out, none of us are permanently "hard wired" at birth. This predetermined conclusion that science has believed for so long is a myth and our understanding of DNA has grown.

One of the pioneers in this field is cell biologist Bruce Lipton, Ph.D., who taught medical students before resigning to do research full-time. In his groundbreaking book called *The Biology of Belief*, Lipton establishes that your mental activity is strong enough to overcome the influences of early conditioning and programming that you unwittingly adopted through your formative years.

In another example of "use-it-or-lose-it" studies were done on Einstein's brain after his death. And yes…his brain was actually different from the average brain. Can you guess in what way, from the list below?

    a.   He had an extra large cerebral cortex.
    b.   His brain weighed one-half pound more than the average brain.
    c.   He had more interconnections among his brain cells.
    d.   He had superior blood flow to the brain.

The correct answer is (c). Studies of Albert Einstein's brain found that the only difference in his brain was that he had developed significantly more nerve cell interconnections than average. What does this mean? Although you can't grow new brain cells…you *can* continue to add new neural connections and brain power for your entire life. Every time you focus and stretch your mind…your brain creates entirely new connections. Literally, the more you use your brain (in certain ways)…the smarter you get!

This means that if we want to change, we can. No excuses! Telling ourselves "I'm too old," or "I'm too young," "I don't know the right people" or "I'm uncoordinated," has no basis in science.

Changing Our Internal Dialogue and Self Talk

We think approximately 60,000 thoughts a day. That means much of our thinking, or self-talk, is subconscious, under-the-radar of our consciousness. Self-talk is a powerful tool that can be either a positive or negative factor in our lives. To make self-talk work in a positive manner we need to make sure it is positive, specific and present tense.

Each of us make choices all day long, with many of these choices being made without our conscious awareness. Whether these choices are to sit in this chair or that chair, what to eat or what to wear, our choices result from our self-talk, an on-going dialogue that we have with ourselves. Very few of these subconscious thoughts even register with our conscious mind, yet they have great influence on our feelings and behaviors. This is why we often find ourselves doing things that we really don't want to do or, conversely, not doing the things that we know we should do.

Positive, specific and present-tense self-talk can overrule self-defeating negative thoughts because our subconscious mind will believe whatever we tell it… if we tell it with conviction. If your conscious self-talk says, "I should clean my desk," or "I ought to clean my desk," then your subconscious mind hears that you are NOT cleaning your desk. As a result, it doesn't move you toward cleaning it.

It's important to know that your subconscious mind sends messages to your motor functions, emotions, and other members of your physical and psychological network. If your subconscious mind believes that you are currently cleaning your desk, then that's what every part of your body will want to be doing.

Let's imagine that you're watching some re-run sitcom on television in which you have little interest. Let's also suppose that while you're watching the show you think that you really should be cleaning your desk. Since your subconscious mind believes what you tell it, if you repeat to yourself, "I am cleaning my desk," then your subconscious mind will focus your attention, physical and mental, on cleaning your desk. Both your body and mind will begin to go into a state of agitation and conflict until you actually go and clean your desk. As long as you repeat your positive, specific, present-tense self-talk message, you will feel compelled to clean your desk.

Your subconscious mind *will* respond to your message. Repeat it over and over and it will respond to your statement.

All the old excuses such as "I'm too busy, I'm too short, too old, not smart enough" can be overruled by dynamic, positive self-talk.

As you will see, *29 DAYS* will help you to use positive self-talk that will help you get past any and all of these old excuses.

> ## *29 DAYS* will help you cut a path through your old thoughts!

Imagine yourself as a forest fireman, whose job it is to set up two observation towers in the middle of a dense tropical forest. You're still in the rainy season and you can practically see the vegetation growing. In every direction all you can see is a wall of green vines, bushes, weeds, plants and trees. You are standing on the spot where you have chosen to erect the first tower. With all the lush growth around, it doesn't take you too long to cut down a number of trees and vines to build the first tower.

With the first tower completed, the real work begins. You need your second tower to be erected, due north, one mile away. This tower has to be built and functional in three weeks before the drier weather brings the inevitable forest fires. Using your machete, you begin to hack a small path through the thick growth. After two weeks of hacking and cutting you finally arrive at the spot where the second tower is to be built, and within a day your second tower is erected.

With both towers set up, your job is to go back and forth between the two towers, twice each day, for observation. As you set out to return to the first tower you can't help but notice that the path you had hacked out is getting thicker and thicker as you make your way back. In fact, aside from the small trees, it looks like it only took about one week for the vegetation to grow back to the thickness it was when you had first cut the trail. Moving a little faster than the first time, you manage to hack your way back through the new growth, and return to the first tower in less than one week.

It is now clear that you have two tasks. The first task is to keep your scheduled observation from each of the two towers, and the second job is to keep the path between the two towers clear enough so that you can quickly travel back and forth between them.

With your quicker return to the first tower, less than one week, you can now return to the second tower in less than two days, since you have quite recently cut down much of the larger growth. Before long you notice that each time you travel between the two towers your speed is increased, and the path is much easier to travel. Within a few days of traveling back and forth the new vegetation doesn't really get a chance to get started. With each trip your feet will crush and press down more of the growth. In fact, the more often you walk this path, the better and easier it becomes. If you travel it four times a day for twenty-nine days in a row it will be a lot more like a roadway than a pathway that somebody hacked into existence with a machete.

Brain scientists have discovered that the same thing happens in your brain when you fire off a thought. You create a new road of neurodes (neuron connections that fire together a thought) when you stimulate your brain by thinking a new thought. Repeating thought patterns strengthens the DSP connections of those patterns and lowers their firing threshold (resistance). Soon these new thoughts become the chosen path to travel.

I can't help but be reminded of Robert Frost's famous poem *The Road Not Taken.*

The Road Not Taken

Two roads diverged in a yellow wood,
And sorry I could not travel both
And be one traveler, long I stood
And looked down one as far as I could
To where it bent in the undergrowth;

Then took the other, as just as fair,
And having perhaps the better claim,
Because it was grassy and wanted wear;
Though as for that the passing there
Had worn them really about the same,

And both that morning equally lay
In leaves no step had trodden black.
Oh, I kept the first for another day!
Yet knowing how way leads on to way,
I doubted if I should ever come back.

I shall be telling this with a sigh
Somewhere ages and ages hence:
Two roads diverged in a wood, and I—
I took the one less traveled by,
And that has made all the difference.

This is the very reason *29 DAYS* courses can be so transformational. Each day you will create new neuron pathways that will soon become a brand new superhighway for your thoughts. Your old thoughts of "I can't lose weight," for example, will quickly become infested with thick brush from lack of travel. The new road of thought such as "What little thing can I do today to help me reach my weight-loss goal?" will become the path that you will begin to mentally travel, and it will happen without effort. You will discover that new empowering thoughts will pop into your head without any conscious effort on your part.

The key to making this happen, and the key to the power of *29 DAYS* courses is simply: repetition, repetition, repetition.

Automate Your Brain for Success – Your Reticular Activating System (RAS)

Brain scientists have discovered an automated system in the brain called the "reticular activating system" (RAS). The RAS is a group of interconnected neurons not located in any specific part of your brain, although it is part of your limbic (subconscious) system.

Every single impulse, whether derived from thought, touch, taste, smell, seeing or hearing, first passes through your RAS.

The RAS then sends signals to the proper area of your brain for interpretation. When something important is on your RAS, it sends a signal to the conscious level for your immediate attention.

Our conscious thought impulses travel about 125 miles per hour. Our subconscious thought impulses travel up to 800 times faster. If someone throws you a baseball and it's heading straight for your face, you don't consciously think: "Okay, I need to tell my hand muscles to open my catching glove, then tell my arm and shoulder muscles to rise up and reach out to catch the ball before it smacks me in the face" If you thought that slowly the ball would have hit you long before you could relay the proper instructions to the various muscles and parts of your body necessary to catch the ball.

One of the most important functions of your RAS is to recognize impulses coming into your brain and determine if it is related to fear, stress, danger, or anxiety. It instantaneously decides if it is something that requires immediate attention or not. If instead of a baseball being thrown at you it was a small child throwing a big plastic beach ball at your face, your RAS may very well choose to ignore it and let it hit you.

If the situation registers as dangerous however, it sends an impulse to your amygdala, which will send another signal out ordering certain hormones and neural transmitters to fire in your brain.

Needless to say this all takes place in a mere fraction of a second.

It is important to remember that your RAS functions at a subconscious level. Another important function of the RAS is that it can be utilized to your conscious benefit. It's the neuroscientific explanation for what the New Thought writers call the *Law of Attraction,* which has received so much attention in the popular book and movie titled *The Secret.*

The Law of Attraction says people's thoughts (both conscious and subconscious) dictate the reality of their lives, whether or not they're aware of it. Essentially, "If you really want something and truly believe it's possible, you'll get it." By the same reasoning, if you put a lot of attention and thought into something you don't want, it means you'll probably get that as well.

Our purpose in *29 DAYS* is not to debate the veracity of the *Law of Attraction,* but rather to point out a simple fact: You will notice that which you put your mind to. *29 DAYS* will very simply help you to keep your mind on your stated objective and goal. Our brain circuits take engrams (memory traces), and produce neuroconnections and neuropathways only if they are bombarded repeatedly (twenty-nine days) without missing a single day!

Have you ever learned a new word and then started to notice that word being used in conversation, on the evening news or in print? Prior to learning that word you probably weren't even aware of its existence.

Suppose you're planning a vacation to an exotic destination. Once again, you will suddenly begin to see ads in magazines, or catch snippets on the news, or overhear people talking about their experience at the very place you're planning to vacation.

If your brain recognizes that something is important to you, your RAS will send that impulse to your conscious level for your immediate attention. If you hold something in mind for a period of time – let's say twenty-nine days, it will be elevated by your RAS to be of paramount importance. If you add emotion to the particular subject of interest, it may well be with you for the rest of your life.

By this reasoning, *29 DAYS* courses will ensure your goals are your RAS's priority.

With this new goal or interest in mind, you will automatically begin to harness the incredible power of your subconscious mind. If you can focus your attention on what you want for twenty-nine days – just by thinking about it, visualizing it, meditating on it, speaking about it and pondering it, you will find solutions, tactics, information and energy coming from seemingly out-of-the-blue. Your subconscious brain will work twenty-four hours a day to help you achieve anything you put your mind to.

Please note, there are certain techniques that are necessary in order to properly set goals and to use visualizing techniques in order to positively harness the power of your subconscious mind. The techniques of visualization, goal setting, written affirmations, etc. and the steps in the *29 DAYS* courses will be discussed in a later section.

— PART FOUR —

The Principles of *29 DAYS*
... to a habit you want!

CHAPTER NINE
The Deceptive Power of Patience and Perseverance

In Chapter Two we said that there are two *Principles of Success:*

Principle #1 is patience and perseverance
Principle #2 is belief and support of our "inner-self."

As we have seen in Part Three, fear is the great obstacle to achieving change. I can think of no better example of the power of taking small steps than the example given by Robert Maurer, Ph.D. in his brilliant book *One Small Step Can Change Your Life*. Dr. Maurer is a practicing psychologist at the UCLA School of Medicine. In this book he tells the story of a woman who is woefully close to the end of her rope, but through his insight and guidance of incremental change she manages to completely transform her life.

Julie had gone to UCLA's medical center for help with high blood pressure and perpetual fatigue. While there she was interviewed by Dr. Mauer and a family practice resident. Julie's story was grim. She was a divorced mother of two who was trying to hold down a job and raise her kids. To add to her challenges she was more than thirty pounds overweight, her job was unsecure, she had no outside support and not surprisingly, she was battling depression.

It was obvious to both doctors that this woman had to make some drastic changes or she was headed for a physical and mental breakdown. When Dr. Mauer looked at the utter despair on Julie's face he knew he had to prescribe something that would actually work rather than what logic might dictate.

Dr. Mauer knew from years of observation, that to suggest she take up an exercise routine, change her diet and try to *will herself* to a healthy lifestyle would actually compound Julie's problems. This is the kind of advice patients like Julie get all the time and the usual result is that they ignore the advice and simply add a guilt trip to their compounding problems.

Surprisingly enough, even when we're living a life of despair and drudgery, familiarity with the life we know offers greater comfort than does change. Change of any kind can cause our most formidable enemy, fear, to to appear.

Julie's life was one of relentless pressure. After a long day at work she would pick-up her kids, drive home, feed them, bath them, put them to bed and then attempt to straighten out the house. Her only break at the end of her day was when she flopped on the couch in utter exhaustion, to watch a half-hour of television before putting herself to bed.

As Dr. Mauer had witnessed on too many occasions, a physician would prescribe an exercise program and the patient, in this case Julie, would think, "Exercise! You have got to be kidding? Do you have any idea what my life is like?"

The physician on the other hand is thinking, "Look, what's the problem here? Don't you care about your body and your health? If you don't do what I prescribe you're heading for serious trouble!"

The biggest problem is a lack of understanding. Julie is totally correct in her thinking because she is convinced she has neither the time, energy or inclination to add an additional half hour of strenuous exercise to her already overloaded day.

The resident with Dr. Mauer was absolutely correct in her assessment and prescribed solution. After all, if a person refuses to take charge of their own health, and lifestyle, then ultimately there's nothing anyone else can do.

Dr. Mauer, however had an 'aha' moment. He knew that he had to try something different in order to break this endless cycle of misery and failure on the part of the physician and the patient.

Just before the inevitable and dreaded aerobics prescription was uttered, Dr. Mauer jumped in and asked Julie if she thought that it might be possible for her to march in front of her television for just *one minute* each day? As the resident looked at him in disbelief, Julie's face actually brightened up and she replied that she could definitely give that a try.

When Julie returned for her follow-up visit she proudly announced that she had faithfully marched in front of her TV set every day for the prescribed sixty seconds. The fact that one minute of exercise would hardly make the slightest dent in affecting Julie's physical health wasn't important at this stage. What was important to Dr. Mauer was that she had actually done it, and she was eager for a slightly bigger challenge. In this short time between her first and second visit, her attitude had noticeably changed and Julie wanted to know what else she could do for sixty seconds a day!

Although it was still early, Dr. Mauer was thrilled with the initial results. Julie had opened her mind to new possibilities. Julie's new challenge was marching for an entire commercial break. Shortly after that, she was marching for two commercial breaks and before long she forgot to stop! Almost without realizing it, Julie had gotten herself to the point of exercising thirty minutes a day and incredibly enough, she was enjoying it!

Within a few months, she was not only embracing the concept of exercise, she was eager to take on full aerobic workouts. Before long she had restored her physical health, her mental health, and her self-esteem.

While working with Julie and other clients in similar situations, Dr. Mauer realized that small, almost embarrassingly trivial steps, were often the solution to dramatic wholesale changes. He realized that getting his patients to buy into the concept (change their fundamental thinking and lay down new neuron tracks) was an essential and crucial first step. Instead of suggesting that a client leave an unfulfilling job, he might ask them to spend a few minutes each day visualizing the "perfect" job. Using this simple, "one-small-step-at-a-time" approach, consistently produced spectacular results.

Dr. Mauer said that a large number of his patients intuitively knew what took him years of observations to conclude: Low-key change helps the human mind to side-step the fear that blocks our ability to achieve our desires. By taking steps that are so small they might seem laughable, we manage to defeat the thoughts of negativity that have always derailed our best intentions in the past.

Minor but consistent effort will cultivate an appetite for success and lay down new ways of thinking and ultimately, permanent results.

The Power of Principle #1

Julie's story is the essence of what *29 DAYS* is all about and why it is so effective. In almost any application, asking someone to march in place for sixty seconds a day would be dismissed as nonsense and an utter waste of time.

In Julie's case, it was probably the only thing that would have worked and the results were nothing short of spectacular.

In *29 DAYS*, we take into consideration that we are all at different stages of development on any given subject. That's why we like to make you your own interactive guide and coach. We will prompt you with a question, give you the proper guidelines in order to correctly answer the question, but ultimately you will come up with a solution that will be just right for you.

Example: Suppose you are the correct weight for your body structure and height, but like Julie, you need to start an exercise program. Our question would be the same to both you and Julie: "What small thing could you do to move you towards an exercise program that you would simultaneously follow and enjoy?" Same question, same guidelines but undoubtedly your answer and Julie's will be quite different.

In Julie's case the answer she may very well have come up with would be to begin by marching in front of the TV for sixty seconds each day. If you were already the correct weight for example, and your time demands weren't as onerous as Julie's, you might suggest that going for a walk in the evening might be just the thing to set you on the path toward beginning an exercise program.

The most important point to take from Julie's story wasn't where she was after thirty days. As anyone can see, marching in place for one minute a day isn't very far along towards establishing a meaningful exercise regimen. And that is precisely when most of us say: "It's no use, nothing is happening." In reality nothing could be further from the truth. On the surface it looked as if Julie hadn't accomplished anything, but below the surface she was establishing a powerful foundation of habit and confidence that wasn't based on the flimsy structure of willpower. After one month Julie had laid down new neuron tracks that were establishing a permanent habit. She was shocked to find herself exercising even when she didn't have to, and within a few short months Julie had graduated to full aerobic workouts!

Our goal in *29 DAYS* is to stay with you and keep your mind engaged and motivated. Keeping you focused for this length of time, while applying small simple tasks, will guarantee that you will step around fear while laying those neuron tracks that are so crucial to forming a lifelong habit. If you faithfully follow the course guidelines, in twenty-nine days your results will be as spectacular as Julie's.

CHAPTER TEN
The Hidden Power of
Support from Our Inner-Self

A True-Life Example of the Power of Principle #2

> You Are a Mirror of Your Inner Thoughts.
> As You See Yourself, So Shall You Be!

In his powerful book, *Over The Top*, Zig Ziglar relates the testimony of a seminar attendee who clearly had a transcending experience. This story is such a wonderful example of the importance of enlisting the support of our inner-self. The central figure in this story was "thin" the moment he *saw himself thin*, even though he had a long way to go to fulfill his goal. (Oops, plot spoiler!)

This story is about a man named Tom who attended one of Zig Ziglar's seminars. At that time he was pretty much down and out. In a letter he wrote to Mr. Ziglar he said that he was recently divorced, he had a job only because the boss was his friend, and at the time he had attended the seminar he weighed over four hundred pounds. He described himself as being financially, morally, spiritually and physically bankrupt; which pretty much covers all bases.

Tom said the seminar had no sooner started when he began to hear a bunch of self-empowering talk about how we can take charge of our lives and how we can change anything we want to change. He considered a quick exit but for one reason or another he ended up staying for the whole day.

As he listened to Mr. Ziglar talk he realized that he had been blaming the negative outcomes of his life on other people and outside circumstances. He was playing the victim-of-fate card. At some point during the day he understood that the moment he began to accept responsibility for his life, he also accepted his *ability to respond*. Tom had an "aha" experience. He finally saw that he had created the mess his life was in, and by extension, he also had the power to turn it around. It was a deep revelation and a moment of instant awakening. At that moment he made up his mind to re-evaluate his life.

The very next day he made some major life changes. He enrolled in a couple of university courses in psychology and joined a health club. At the end of the week he went to a clothing store and put a small downpayment on a bunch of clothes that would fit his body type if he weighed two hundred pounds less!

Tom said he was at last committed to change and the most significant thing he did was to *see himself* as a new person. He knew his new image of himself was complete when he caught himself staring at a store's front window one day. While he was absorbing the goods on display he saw a reflection in the window of some big guy standing right behind him. He spun around to see who it was and to his surprise there was no one there. Tom had simply seen his own reflection in the window, which he no longer recognized.

The reason that little episode is of such monumental importance is that Tom had made a complete transformation from the hopeless person who had attended the seminar just a few weeks earlier. Although he still weighed over three hundred and eighty pounds, he no longer *saw* himself as an obese person. He had changed the way he saw himself and the way he thought. He now saw himself at his ideal weight. At that point he said he knew, "and he knew that he knew" he was going to make it. What he was really saying is that he *saw his future.*

Tom had taken responsibility for his life, and because he was in control, he knew that no force on earth could stop him from achieving his goals.

In Tom's case he visualized himself as a new person. He saw himself in a new light. He saw a person who enjoyed total physical, spiritual, financial and emotional health. Within a short period of time, he had graduated with his degree in psychology and he began working on his doctorate. He eventually brought his weight down to just a little over two hundred pounds which is where it should be since he stands 6′ 3″ and has a large frame.

Tom changed his thoughts and the results were nothing short of extraordinary.

The Power of Principle #2

It was of particular interest to note that even when Tom weighed over 380 pounds, he *saw* himself as thin. At this point his goal, to lose the rest of the weight, was a *fait accompli.*

Once he had changed the way he saw himself (created new neural pathways of thought) nothing could stop his inevitable victory. He had effectively harnessed the power of his inner-self ... his conscious and subconscious mind.

Tom's mental makeover was much like Julie's in the previous story. Although Julie had physically accomplished very little in the first month, she had changed her thinking (new neural pathways) which led to greater and greater activity until within a few short months she was engaged in full aerobic activity. What Julie and Tom accomplished in the first month through patience, perseverance and the support of their inner-self, was everything they needed to carry them to their ultimate goals.

This is the essence of the power of *29 DAYS*. Our goal is not to look to the top of the mountain, which is our ultimate goal, but rather to focus on what we can do in the very short term that will build a highway to our desired achievement.

Picture yourself standing on a hilltop overlooking a series of neighboring hills. Since it's a beautiful day and you're in the mood for hiking, you decide to scale the nearby hill since it's only a mile or so away. As you descend the hill and begin to cross the valley, you get a sense that this new hill is somewhat further away than you had originally anticipated. In fact, it seems like it might be several miles farther than you had first thought. At this point what would you logically conclude? That you're *farther away* from the new hill than when you started or that you are making progress but it will take longer than you expected?

This is a most common scenario many of us experience when facing a new challenge or goal. We often misjudge what will be required, but then make a further mistake and assume that after weeks or months of effort, we're actually further away from our goal than when we started. But, like the hiker, we *have to* be making progress even though it may not initially appear to be so. When we find ourselves at this point of doubt, it's imperative that we keep our focus on the next task at hand, rather than looking at the top of the distant hill and concluding that it's actually moving away from us.

A great analogy to keep in mind is when you're driving your car at night. Your headlights will allow you to see only a few hundred feet in front of you, but that has no bearing on how far you can travel. You may travel as far as you wish without ever seeing more than a few hundred feet ahead.

29 DAYS strives to keep you focused on the immediate task at hand, because if you can do this without getting discouraged, your big goals will fall into place far easier and quicker than you will have dreamed possible.

— <u>PART FIVE</u> —

Bringing It All Together

CHAPTER ELEVEN
How *29 DAYS* Will Help You To Achieve Your Goals in an Effortless Way

Tools and Techniques for Permanent Change

As we stated in the Introduction, all of us are mirror reflections of our self image; our thoughts, fears, beliefs and attitudes. If we cannot change those things, we cannot instill "lasting" change.

The reason positive change is often so difficult can be reduced to two basic human traits:

1. When we attempt to change something about ourselves, we want change to happen immediately, and if we don't see it immediately, we often give up and assume whatever technique we were trying simply doesn't work. We overlook the vital requisite of patience and persistence.

2. We try to change too much too soon through sheer force of will. Before long we find that we cannot sustain the requisite energy at that heightened level. We quickly get discouraged and return to our former ways.

The tools we will use to achieve success such as; *How to Write a Goal, Visualization, Asking Small Questions, Written Affirmations, Granting Ourselves Small Rewards*, and *Taking Small Steps*, work so well because they are strung together in a way that is effective without being overbearing.

29 DAYS courses can actually be everything that a hired coach can be and more for several reasons. It is very often human nature to want to do things by ourselves and for ourselves. Sometimes that can be good, and sometimes it can lead to frustration and capitulation. Have you ever had to fill out a form for a bank account or a mortgage application? If you have, you know what an unpleasant task that can be. "When were you born?" "Where do you live?" "What's your driver's license number?" … and on and on. Have you also had the experience of having to fill out a the same type of form but instead of you doing it all on your own, you had someone else ask you the questions and then fill in the responses for you? In this case you're still coming up with the same answers, but with someone else helping it seems so much easier. I don't know if it's because there are two people doing it, or if it's just more comfortable not to have to do it yourself, but with someone else's prompting the task seems almost effortless.

In our courses we want you to enjoy the same experience. We will prompt you with a question, along with the proper way to frame an answer, and you simply respond.

This Sounds Like a One-Size-Fits-All Solution!

Definitely not! It's true that questions we ask will be the same to each participant, but the answers and responses to those questions are personal to you. Each response will be as unique to you as your fingerprints. The process of setting goals and asking the right questions are universal. The answers you supply are not.

Your Personal Coach in *29 DAYS* is the *most supportive coach in the world!* How couldn't he/she be, it's ultimately YOU! In addition to being totally supportive to your success, your enrollment in this course can be kept as confidential as you wish.

The Importance of Privacy

Although it's completely up to you, the fact that you can take a course in complete privacy can also be an important factor toward achieving your desired results. In the case of Julie, if she had told anyone (including her amygdala) what she was working toward, she would have been ridiculed remorselessly. You can just hear the negative comments about the foolishness of sixty seconds of marching. At this early stage we may be very vulnerable and susceptible to the negative influence of others. Keeping our goals and our program to ourselves until we establish those strong inner beliefs, can be integral to our success.

CHAPTER TWELVE
How To Set a Goal, Visualizing a Goal

Earl Nightingale once wrote, "Happiness is the progressive realization of a worthy goal."

You feel truly happy when you are making progress, step-by-step. When you're absolutely clear about your goal, you do not have to know how you're going to achieve it. By simply deciding exactly what you want, you will begin to move unerringly toward your goal, and your goal will start to move unerringly toward you. At exactly the right time and in exactly the right place, you and your goal will meet.

> *Give me a stock clerk with a goal, and I will give you a man who will make*
> *history. Give me a man without a goal, and I will give you a stock clerk.*
> ~ *J.C. Penney*

Your written goals must be described in a positive, personal tense.

Let's suppose your goal is to lose thirty pounds. *(As we said initially, we would use weight loss for our examples but this is the exact same process for saving money, quitting smoking, etc.)* Using the philosophy of *29 DAYS*, you're going to set a goal that you absolutely *know* you can achieve in twenty-nine days. Remember, your ultimate goal is much bigger than what you can accomplish in twenty-nine days. In fact, your goal is much bigger than losing the thirty pounds per se. Your real goal is to program yourself to enjoy a lifetime of health and inner-self-confidence without ever having to worry about your weight and what you eat again.

Your *29 DAYS* course goal might be to lose five pounds, and your lifetime goal might be to enjoy perfect health at your ideal weight of let's say 155 pounds. You now have an immediate goal and a lifetime goal.

Activate Your Subconscious Mind

29 DAYS will strive to keep you focused on your goal, not the process.

When a goal states exactly what it is you want to be, have or do, it then becomes easy to communicate precise details of your desire to your subconscious.

In his book *The Path of Least Resistance*, Robert Fritz talks about learning to become the creative force in your own life. On choosing to be the creative force he writes that many people get lost in the process. They spend their time and energy focusing on all the stuff they associate with getting to their goal rather than focusing on the goal itself. He writes:

> *Many people engaged in processes designed to bring them specific results have never actually chosen those results, either formally or informally. Some people who eat special health foods, take large doses of vitamin supplements, exercise assiduously, and avoid alcohol, coffee, tobacco, chocolate, bleached flour, red meat, and refined sugar have never made the choice to be healthy. Many people take healthful actions and still do not make the choice to be healthy.*

In other words, we often get so caught up in the process we forget to set our mission. Picture someone who decides to go on a diet in order to lose weight. Very often they dive into the program with reckless abandon and the probable result will be failure. Why? Their focus will be entirely on the process. They begin with an austerity program. They limit themselves to making, eating or ordering certain foods. They cut back on other foods. They focus on counting calories. They're thinking about their food intake all day long. They're totally focused on successfully completing the diet or losing the twenty, thirty or forty pounds. In order to speed-up the process they may even resort to exercising for a few weeks. Each meal becomes a major issue. They talk about it, moan about it and tell everyone the latest details. Can you see the holes in this process? Can you see how utterly unsustainable this is?

Have you ever seen someone who is busy from morning to night but never seems to accomplish anything? They're those frazzled, harried people who rush around with a slight scowl because life is always just out of reach. In many ways that is a mirror reflection of someone who dives into a process. What happens after they lose the weight? What happens when the process is completed? The person caught-up in this typical scenario fails to ask the big question; "And then what?"

If people would focus on an outcome, rather than a diet, the entire process takes on a radically different appearance. The procedure is more cerebral, more relaxed, more definite and ultimately sustainable. Making the choice for health and your perfect weight will gather the inner resources of the body, mind, and spirit. Using this method you and the unseen forces begin to work toward a mutual meeting ground. You align the energies toward your desire.

This is where the power of visualizations and affirmations and the subconscious forces come to your aid.

There are two ways to think about goals. You can write a goal for your conscious mind and you can also create a goal for your subconscious mind. There is a difference.

Conscious Mind Goals

Your conscious mind thinks in terms of time; past, present and future. If your goal is to lose thirty pound then a clearly written, conscious goal might be written like this;

I weigh 155 pounds on x date. This is a goal that is written in a positive tense with a specific time.

Subconscious Mind Goals

Your subconscious mind has no concept of time. It only functions in the present. Therefore when you communicate with your subconscious mind you will do so in the form of an affirmation. A goal for your conscious mind written as: "I weigh 155 pounds on x date," would become an affirmation to your subconscious mind that you would repeat as: "I weigh 155 pounds." The only difference is that you don't put a date on it. You relay this desire to your subconscious mind and it will find a way to achieve your goal.

You put the date on it for your conscious mind so that it becomes a believable goal for you. This aligns the believability your conscious mind needs to the positive, emotional feeling that fuels your subconscious mind.

As noted earlier, our subconscious mind is our success tool. Unfortunately we were never taught how to use it effectively. If you wish to eliminate a bad habit it is imperative to write your goal in a positive/positive way. In each of the courses we will walk with you step by step toward the proper way of writing and setting your goals.

Why Do You Want this Goal?

What is your purpose? What will achieving this goal do for you? What will it do for the way you feel, your self-confidence? How will it positively effect those around you? Will your increased confidence put you in a better state of mind, allowing you to be a better person to be around? Will it it effect your finances, your relationships?

You will think of many positive ways to achieve your goal. This exercise will give you enduring motivation. To succeed at anything, it's vital to know why you are doing whatever it is you are doing.

Are There Any Downsides to Achieving Your Goal?

Now is the time to be aware of any downsides to achieving your goals. You don't want to be well into achieving your goal only to have your amygdala, or inner-demons, come up with an excuse at the last possible moment in order to upset all the progress you've made.

If you know in advance of any "tricks" that might come up, and they will, you can address them as old news that's already been considered and dismiss these thoughts with a "Nice-try-but-it-won't-work" response.

Every time you write your goals or express your affirmations, you are impressing them deeper and deeper into your subconscious mind. At a certain point, you will begin to believe, with absolute conviction, that your goal is achievable. Once your subconscious mind accepts your goals as commands from your conscious mind, it will start to make all your words and actions fit a pattern consistent with those goals. Your subconscious mind will start attracting people and circumstances into your life that can help you to achieve your goal. Be clear about your goal, but be flexible about the process of achieving it.

In the *29 DAYS* courses we will reach out to you twice each day with tips, inspiring information, stories, encouragement – in short, all the things a good coach does. When you hear from us will depend on when you check your email. Reading your morning message is often the perfect time to spend thirty seconds reviewing your goal. If you review your goal twice a day, you will quickly create new neural pathways, new beliefs.

The more you review your goal, the larger, stronger and more often these neuron patterns will fire. These neuron patterns are new beliefs programmed into your subconscious by choice. Brain research has proven that neural pathways, used often, create the largest neuron patterns and fire the easiest. Stated another way, the more you think about something, the easier it is to think about it over and over again. This is how many of us have unwittingly reinforced our own negative behavior.

States of Mind

In order to access your subconscious mind most effectively you need to be aware of your various states of mind. The four states of mind are Beta, Alpha, Theta and Delta. Each of these states is distinguished by brain waves, which are determined by the amount of mental activity. When we are in our normal awake state we are in 'beta' which is characterized by a brain wave frequency of 14 to 35 cps (cycles per second). The beta state is by far the most erratic because it is constantly evaluating everything that is going on around us. This awareness is essential for conducting our daily affairs and our general survival.

The alpha state is characterized by a brain wave frequency of 8 to 13 cps. You naturally go into the alpha state a number of times during the day, but usually for only brief periods. You know you have been in the alpha state when you catch yourself daydreaming or staring off into space. I used to catch myself dwelling in the alpha state for long stretches of time when I was at church or school. The alpha state is referred to as the "meditative" state – a state of relaxed, focused concentration.

The theta state (4 to 7 cps) is similar to the alpha state but deeper and characterized by sudden intuitive insights or the "super learning" brain state. The theta is the brain state you were often in up to about six years of age. This is when the subconscious accepts and records everything without any filtering. This is why we often do things or behave in certain ways as adults that can seem inexplicable to us. These bizarre behaviors can often be attributed to early programing by parents, siblings, teachers and television long before we were consciously aware of it, and certainly before we were capable of filtering out the unwanted stuff.

The last state is the delta state (3cps and lower.) This is the sleep state in which there is no consciousness. Dreaming occurs in the alpha and theta states.

It is important to be aware of these various states of mind if you wish to have a greater influence on your subconscious mind and to be able to change your way of thinking.

You may have heard of the various studies that have been done on Indian fakirs or the participants in the annual *Phuket Vegetarian Festival,* where they are able to change their heart rates, body temperature or push unsterilized swords and spears through their bodies. There are dozens of grotesque but fascinating pictures on the internet showing the vegetarian devotees with various objects pushed through their cheeks and yet they're immune to infection and their wounds heal rapidly without leaving a single mark.

To achieve these amazing feats requires the participants to be in an altered state of mind. In order for them to control involuntary body functions they had to be in the alpha or theta states. Thus, the alpha and theta brain wave states are the doorways to your subconscious mind.

Suggestions and commands to your subconscious mind are least effective when your mind is in the beta state where your conscious mind dominates. Your subconscious mind however, will accept suggestions and commands much more readily when you are in the alpha and theta states. This is why affirmations and visualizations are so effective just when you are about to fall asleep or when you first wake up. Knowing that your subconscious is so receptive while in the alpha or theta state, repeating affirmations when in these states will focus your mind to fire with thought patterns reflective of your affirmations.

Incidently, the advertising industry is acutely aware of this phenomenon. When you're watching television do you have a tendency to let your mind go blank during commercials? You may actually pay attention to a commercial the first or second time you see it, but after repeated exposure you begin to consciously tune it out. Make no mistake, advertisers would much rather have you in this "tune-out" state (alpha) because then they are tapping straight into your subconscious mind. When you're in the beta state you might even think ... "What a ridiculous commercial! Who could possibly believe that?" The answer, your subconscious, that's who. That is precisely why advertisers will hit you with the same commercial over and over and over in a single show. They don't care what you consciously think, they want to lay down those powerful neuron tracks in your subconscious.

It's also not a bad idea to enjoy periodic daydreaming about things you desire and goals you wish to achieve. When you are in these receptive states (alpha states) you are super charging your subconscious.

When you first awaken each day, the subconscious is in the "alpha" or learning state and is most susceptible to re-programming. Then throughout the day your subconscious will bring to your attention anything which draws you closer to achieving your goals. At night while you sleep, your subconscious is still awake and active. What you focus on immediately before bed is what your subconscious will work on. Reviewing your goals before bed gives you the extra advantage of having your subconscious mind work on achieving your goals while you sleep.

This is why many psychologists recommend you do not watch the news before bed. Your subconscious will constantly be focused on events like war, murder or terrorism, negativity.

Your subconscious mind works like a massive computer that is never turned off. It will work tirelessly to bring you whatever it is that you focus on. Once your subconscious is locked on target, almost without your doing anything, it will materialize your dominant thought. Negative thoughts bring negative results. Focus on your goals and they will begin to materialize in your life, sometimes in the most remarkable and unexpected ways.

The belief that you cannot have what you want
creates a tension that is resolved by not having what you want.
~ Robert Fritz

Visualize Your Goal for Ultimate Success

"Imagination is more important than knowledge"
~ Albert Einstein

Visualization and Your Subconscious Mind

Your mind and a computer have one thing in common: neither of them know the
difference between the truth ... and what you tell it.
~ Ken Blanchard

Visualization can be such a powerful mental tool because we can literally create the experience we desire if the actual one we need is not available. Through our imagination and visualization, we can create the experience synthetically. Science has proven that the human nervous system is incapable of distinguishing between actual experience and the same experience imagined vividly and in complete detail.

Worry is a perfect example of how we create the synthetic experience. When we worry about something what are we actually doing? We are projecting ourselves mentally, emotionally and even physically into a situation that hasn't even occurred!

If you think visualization doesn't work, let's consider the following. Have you personally, or do you know of anyone who worried so intensely about something that they've actually managed to make themselves sick? The fact is, if a person worries intensely enough about failure he will experience the same reactions that accompany actual failure. He will experience feelings of anxiety, humiliation, and before long, headaches and ulcers. As far as his mind and body are concerned he has failed.

If you think about it, worry is the *negative use* of creative imagination and visualization. It simply cannot be anything else. Worry is nothing but a vividly imagined negative synthetic experience. It can't be anything other than synthetic because it hasn't happened!

The man who worries about failure is unknowingly defeating himself through negative feelings and emotions. He's feeding himself negative data. If he spent the same amount of time *visualizing* success he would invariably *produce* success. Instead of heartburn and ulcers, he could deliberately mold the life he desires.

Each of us, whether we realize it or not, constantly practice visualization and self actualization. Why not practice visualizing the person you most want to become? This is the person you *can* become. Use your spare moments to concentrate on your goals. Put more into the positive use of your imagination rather than devoting energy into worry. It really is that simple. Show me a worry-wart that achieves success. He doesn't achieve success, but he *does* achieve his outcome. The process works, one hundred percent, every time. In 29 DAYS, that is exactly what you will do. You will concentrate and focus on the exact outcome you desire.

Each of us is the product of all our thoughts and experiences. Through thought, we can control, to an almost unbelievable degree, both our experience and environment. Whether we choose to direct our own course through life or not is entirely up to us. The important thing is to know it can be done.

Visualize Your Goal Continually

Visualization takes advantage of the latest neuroscience discoveries that suggest that the brain learns best not in large dramatic steps, but instead in very small increments. These small steps are likely a lot smaller than you've probably even imagined!

You possess and have available to you virtually unlimited mental powers. Many people are unaware of these powers and fail to use them for goal attainment. Your ability to visualize is perhaps the most powerful faculty that you possess. All improvements in your life begin with an improvement in your mental pictures.

Visualization activates the *Law of Attraction*, which draws into your life the people, circumstances, and resources that you need to achieve your goals. As it happens, you are always visualizing something, one way or another. Every time you think of someone or something, remember a past event, imagine an upcoming event, or even daydream, you are visualizing. Visualization is simply self-talk that uses mental pictures rather than words. It is essential that you learn to manage and control this visualizing capability of your mind and focus it like a laser beam.

Things to remember

- Your subconscious cannot tell the difference between truth and a lie, reality or imagination. This is why you can look in the mirror, see your overweight image but still say "I am fit and slim."

  Even if your conscious brain says B.S., your subconscious goes to work to create the "fit and slim" you.

- Your subconscious sees in pictures, images and patterns.

- Actions always come from the images (pictures) you create in your mind.

- The more you send an image down a neural pathway the clearer, easier and quicker it fires in the order you have visualized.

- Strong emotion attached to any visualization increases the ease in which your neurode pattern fires.

- It takes twenty-one to twenty-eight days to create a new habit.

A Real World Example of the Power of Visualization

As we mentioned earlier, Dr. Maxwell Maltz, M.D., wrote the timeless classic, *Psycho-Cybernetics*, in which he concluded that a person's actions, feelings, behaviors, and even abilities, are consistent with his or her self-image. In other words, you will become the sort of person you think and see yourself being. Change your vision and you will change yourself.

Dr. Maltz told the story of the time he was working with an ex-convict who was desperately trying to turn his life around. The man explained to Dr. Maltz that he felt magnetically drawn to frequent his old hangouts, but by doing so he knew he was playing with dynamite. Not only were his old friends a bad influence, but hanging with them was a direct violation of his parole conditions. Although the ex-con tried his best to avoid the usual people and places, at a deeper level he said he felt that this was just his lot in life. He was just cut-out to be a lowlife convict Dr. Maltz explained to him that if decided to think that; "I'm just a loser" or "I am what I am," he might just as well pack his up his kit because he was heading straight back to jail.

Dr. Maltz told the man that if he truly wanted to break his old thought patterns about being a loser who was destined for jail, that he should make two simple drawings. They could be stick figure drawings for all it mattered, but the man was instructed to draw one picture of himself standing in a jail cell and a sign above the door that read, *"That's Just The Way I am Prison."* The other drawing was to show a man walking away from the prison toward his family. The caption on the second picture was to read; *"I am what I decide to be."*

Dr. Maltz then told the man to make a few copies of these pictures and put them in places where he would see them for the next several weeks. He was to put them in his locker at work, his lunch pail, his car etc. so he would be constantly reminded of his options and direction in life. Each time he looked at the pictures he was to envision the life he desired.

Before long the man told Dr. Maltz that the two simple picture drawings had actually "drove him sane." Each time he thought of heading out to the pub to see his old friends the pictures and thoughts of his family flooded his mind. Before long he was pulled in only one direction, home.

After just one month the urge to associate with his delinquent buddies had all but disappeared. He had begun to make new thought patterns and new ways of thinking.

"I can zero in on a vision of where I want to be in the future. I can see it so clearly in front of me, when I daydream, it's almost a reality. Then I get this easy feeling, and I don't have to be uptight to get there because I already feel like I'm there, that it's just a matter of time."

"I set a goal, visualize it very clearly, then create the drive, the hunger for turning it into a reality. There's a kind of joy in that kind of ambition, in having a vision in front of you. With that kind of joy, discipline isn't difficult or negative or grim. You love doing what you have to do – going to the gym, working hard on the set. Even when pain is part of reaching your goal, and it usually is, you can accept that too."
~ Arnold Schwarzenegger

Remember, whatever you focus on is what
the subconscious believes you want.
What it believes you want, you'll get!

CHAPTER THIRTEEN
The Power of Focused Repetition

A habit is something that we do repeatedly and often without effort. Now, if only all of our habits were good ones! In order to create the good habits we want, we need to be sure our thoughts are consistently focused on what we want.

The *29 DAYS* courses will ensure that your thoughts stay focused on your goal. As for the rest … the laws of attraction and universal intelligence will play their part.

Affirmations

Before I understood how the subconscious mind receives and responds to our conscious thoughts, I thought affirmations and visualization to be nothing more than a bunch of New Age garbage.

The reality is that your subconscious mind *did* get programmed, and much of that programming went on before you were ever aware of it. In fact, most of the beliefs that you hold have been put there by someone or something else *without* your knowledge or permission.

So exactly how was this programming installed?

Excellent question and glad you asked. It was presented by outside influence (parents, teachers, television, friends) and installed by your subconscious awareness through the tools of affirmation and visualization.

We need to simply use the same method but install the programs of *our conscious choice* instead. It's that simple. So please do not think of affirmations and visualization as New Age hype, it's very real and very effective.

What exactly are affirmations and how do we make them work?

Affirmations are statements that you repeat to your subconscious brain to help you make positive changes. Affirmations are often viewed with a great deal of skepticism, because we have a tendency to think of affirmations as someone running about screaming "I am great, I am great," but that's a limited view. Our belief system is nothing short of a series of visualizations and affirmations.

If you give your subconscious new affirmations you begin to create new DSP connections (see Chapter Eight) in your brain that change, or at least overwrite, the beliefs and attitudes that were installed from previous "unwanted" affirmations.

A technique that is recommended by researchers in the field of brain science is to repeat an affirmation while looking into a mirror because a mirror generates emotion. When you generate emotion, you create stronger, longer-lasting neuron connections. Even if you know consciously that what you're affirming is false, it *will* generate emotion.

Suppose you wish to lose thirty pounds. If you stand in front of your mirror and say; "I am fit and trim," your conscious mind might be screaming B.S., but your subconscious mind says "okay."

Your subconscious mind will begin to go into action to create a fit and trim you. If you're skeptical about this technique, and many people are, don't forget, you are the result of your thoughts. So ask yourself, where did my thoughts and beliefs come from? Can you recall the time that you sat down and said to yourself? "You know, I think I would like to be overweight." Of course not, but here you are (assuming you're overweight). Whatever your thoughts and habits are, they had to come from somewhere!

Throughout the *29 DAYS* course, and through the morning and evening interaction with you, you will find yourself repeatedly and effortlessly thinking about your goal, even if it's only a silent affirmation.

Each day you will be engaging the highly effective method of building new neural connections in your brain. Through the power of focus and repetition your mind will enthusiastically take over the process of change. With this concerted inner-support, you will be astonished at the ease and rapidity you make towards achieving your goal.

Character is not a thing of chance, but the result of continued focus. In fact it's the result of many unconscious affirmations. The easiest and most natural way to change an unwanted character trait is to select an affirmation which seems to fit your particular case. The positive thought will destroy the negative as certainly as light destroys darkness, and the results will be just as effective.

As stated earlier, we are the sum total of our thoughts. So if that is the case, how can we initiate so many good thoughts that they literally crowd out the bad? We actually can't stop the bad thoughts from coming but when they arrive we don't have to play host and entertain them. By using a ready-made positive affirmation we can begin to push the negative thoughts out. When a thought of anger, jealousy, fear or worry creeps in, just start up a counteractive affirmation.

The way to eliminate darkness is with light. The way to eliminate cold is with heat. The way to overcome evil is with good. When unwanted thoughts pop into your mind, simply affirm a positive affirmation and the bad thoughts will vanish.

And you shall decree a thing,
and it will be given unto you.
And light will shine upon your ways.
~ Job 22:28

CHAPTER FOURTEEN
The Power of Awareness

29 DAYS employs written goals, visualization and focused repetition. Each of these are powerful influencers in generating the forces to help us achieve our goals. Another tool in the drawer is how *29 DAYS* will keep you constantly aware of your goal, magically harnessing hidden, and inexplicable forces.

A recent Harvard University Study, published in a 2007 issue of *Psychological Science* tracked the health of eighty-four female room attendants working in seven different hotels.

The study found that those who recognized their work as exercise experienced significant health benefits. Cleaning hotel rooms is a physically taxing job. Each woman scours a hotel room for twenty to thirty minutes, cleaning an average of fifteen rooms a day.

The women were separated into two groups, one learned how their work fulfilled the recommendations of daily activity levels while the other, control group, went about work as usual.

Although neither group changed its behavior, the women who were conscious of their activity level experienced a significant drop in weight, blood pressure, body fat, waist to hip ratio and body mass index in just four weeks. The control group experienced no improvements despite engaging in the exact same physical activities.

The study illustrates how profoundly a person's attitude can affect ones physical well being and by extension, anything else we are focused on.

> Remember whatever you focus on
> is what the subconscious believes you want.

CHAPTER FIFTEEN
The Power of Questions

Anytime that you ask yourself a question you will get an answer. Which is why it is imperative that we ask ourselves positive, empowering questions. Our brains love to respond to challenges, and questions are challenges that request an answer.

If you ask yourself: "Why is my life so disorganized?," your brain might reply; "It's because you're a lazy slob!" *That* is not an empowering question. Suppose you changed the question to: "What small thing can I do to bring organization into my life?" Now you are beginning to ask a question that will bring you a positive, empowering answer.

> We thrive on questions, not directives.

Whether a set of directives come from an authority figure, a book, a course, or ourselves, we will have a natural tendency to resist. When faced with directives we have a natural tendency to either tune them out or deeply resist them.

A series of innocuous questions will usually achieve the exact result we desire — an answer and a solution to our query that will be uniquely tailored to our own personal situation.

Using weight loss as our example, if you were to ask, "What small thing could I do today to lose weight?," the answer that you come up with will be perfectly suited to you. The answers you might come up with might be to substitute a piece of fruit for a slice of pie. You might say, "I'll take that elevator to one floor short of my destination and walk the last flight of stairs." You might say, "I'll take a parking spot at the far end of the lot and not only save my car from the inevitable dings and dents, but I'll enjoy the extra walk." It doesn't matter what the situation is, if you ask yourself, "What small thing could I do?" you will be amazed at the wonderful and creative answers your brain will supply.

These small steps are the secret elixir, the magic of achievement! Consider this: If you gain ten pounds a year, within ten years you are obese, but incredibly you may only be overeating by an average of less than one hundred calories a day. That amounts to little more than a tablespoon of oil, a third of a candy bar, or half a handful of peanuts. In point of fact then, packing on excess weight can happen in the most innocuous manner, and by the same logic, a tiny adjustment in the opposite direction will bring the weight down in the exact same way.

A Re-Cap of the Five Simple Steps

Step One

☞ Each day, for twenty-nine days, you will find yourself thinking about your goal. Far too often people work on a daily goal, and actually make measurable progress, but fail to notice, or recognize their achievement. A simple acknowledgement of achievement will reinforce your inner self-confidence allowing success to build upon success.

Step Two

☞ Each course will supply you with a visual measuring system to chart your daily progress. The program will allow you to choose an inspiring picture (from our library or preferably one of your own). On day one, when we begin, your picture will serve as a visual image that will help you to see your daily progress. Let's suppose it's a picture of a mountain. Each day when you have completed your simple task, you will respond to the *29 DAYS* course which will indicate that you have completed the day's request. This response will simply require you to click on a live "send" URL button, and we will be able to confirm your simple Action Step. When we receive your response, we will send you 1/29th of your picture in your evening message. Each day you will be sent another piece of the picture to serve as a visual reference toward the attainment of your goal. As you see more and more of the picture being completed, it will serve to stimulate your confidence and serve as an external mirror to the internal development of your desired goal. With each successive day your confidence will grow. Success breeds success until it will seem almost effortless.

Step Three

☞ *29 DAYS* courses give you the aid of daily support. Any athlete will tell you that accountability automatically improves performance. Just the act of reporting your progress to someone is helpful to staying on track. Very often we may want to keep our goals confidential. The program's interaction with you is restricted to interaction between you and your online coach. You will enjoy complete anonymity.

Step Four

☞ *29 DAYS* courses ensure that you reward yourself for your progress. So often we are so stuck with our noses to the grindstone that we wear ourselves out. Even though we are making positive progress we wind up feeling like failures. You can build your confidence by acknowledging and celebrating your small victories on a daily or weekly basis. Every seven days is marked with a reward that is the most effective of psychological motivators known.

Step Five

☞ Avoid getting burned out. *29 DAYS* is a powerful tool that ensures you avoid burnout. Together we will make certain that you are continually making forward progress, but at a pace that is both easy, measurable and enjoyable.

CHAPTER SIXTEEN
How Our Changing Wants and Desires Might Apply in the Real World

Keeping with our examples of weight loss, let's suppose you just love going to McDonald's, KFC or some other fast-food restaurant. Let's further suppose that you find yourself visiting "Ronald" or the "Colonel" twice a week, or eight times a month. Do you think that if you were to reduce your visits to oh, say, seven times a month, that it would make you feel greatly deprived? Highly unlikely!

Now the point is this. Let's say that during the course of one month you skipped just *one* visit to the Colonel and by visiting him just six times that month, instead of seven, it didn't leave you feeling the least bit deprived. Now suppose two months later you cut your visit to six times per month and so on until a year or two from now these "quick fix" outlets no longer even register on your radar. Your life and lifestyle in this area would have totally changed.

This new lifestyle is not about being a crusader, it's not about converting anyone else, or bad mouthing fast-food restaurants. It's simply a quiet change of desire that will be with you for the rest of your life. In fact, if you happened to go to a fast-food restaurant because you were out with a bunch of friends and that's where you ended up, so be it. You can eat a small portion, or choose something a little more healthful, *or not*, but now it's a once-in-a-blue-moon situation that will have almost no effect on your total health. The point is this, whether it's fast-food restaurants or some other weight-challenging problem, in a year or two from now you can see how easily you can change your lifestyle with a little focused thought and simple awareness, and, most importantly, you wouldn't feel the least bit deprived.

That is what permanent and lasting change is all about! And, it only takes twenty-nine days for you to think quite differently.

Now, if we can stack six or seven other small changes, such as drinking enough water, or enjoying a piece of fruit as much as an ice cream bar, then "suddenly" within a few months from now you will have a very different lifestyle. In fact, you will have magically changed your life in this area without teeth-gritted will-power. You will have simply started making different choices, and most rewarding is that these choices will have been made from an effortless point of "conscious awareness."

CHAPTER SEVENTEEN
There are No Shortcuts ... but *29 DAYS* Can Happen Surprisingly Quickly

In the *29 DAYS* courses we ask only two things – that you stay with this course for the entire duration and that you actively participate each day. We promise that if you do, you will be blown away by the results.

> Nothing of any value or meaning happens instantly.
> Everything worthwhile involves a process.

- Picture yourself as an electronics salesperson at a stereo shop. A customer walks into your store and says "I'm here to buy a complete stereo system for my recreation room. I have $4,000 to spend." You've got a luncheon appointment and you're pressed for time so instead of asking questions about the type of music he listens to and the size of the room etc. you reply; "You're in luck. We have just the equipment you need," and you start writing up the bill. Do you suppose the customer will hand over his $4,000 just like that? Highly unlikely. What is more probable is that you've blown an easy sale.

- Tammy's a young teenager who has a mad crush on her high school's star athlete. She is certain that her life would be utterly complete if only he would only ask her to be his date at the upcoming graduation dance. Then to Tammy's complete joy, he calls and asks her out to a movie. The next evening they go to a drive-in and Tammy's date tries to kiss her within the first twenty minutes. Tammy gets spooked and jumps out of the car.

- A world-class speed skater decides to "take-up" downhill skiing. She goes to the mountain and asks for some lessons from the resident ski instructor. She and the instructor start off on the bunny-hill where she is shown the basics of how to turn and how to stop. She quickly grows tired of the tedium and details and decides to ride the ski lift to the top of the mountain. Once there she chooses to go down a black diamond (a very difficult run) slope and she gets seriously injured.

- It's the second day of January, and aside from a slight hangover, Isaac is feeling ready to go. He's committed to fulfilling his New Year's resolution to pack on some muscle and lose some weight. Isaac goes to the gym for the first time in many years. He wants to get fit and trim as quickly as possible so he spends four hours pumping weights. The next day Isaac can't get out of bed, and on top of that, he's managed to pull a muscle.

Although these are just made-up situations, you can be sure that the world is chock full of stories just like these. Everything in life requires a process – whether we like it or not. If we can curb our desires for instant gratification we can have just about anything we can set our minds to, and we can usually attain it far easier than we ever imagined.

Enjoying life and achieving our goals doesn't have to be difficult. As we said in the very beginning, it's all in the way we look at a thing.

CHAPTER EIGHTEEN
How Often Do We Play the Martyr?

I love the example that Zig Ziglar gives in his book *See You At The Top* about the pain, and sacrifice he went through while losing weight and getting physically fit. He tells about the "enormous price" he had to pay every morning by getting out of a warm bed into the cold and discomfort of running through his neighborhood. Since he traveled a great deal he would belly-ache endlessly about running in the heat of California or the cold of Winnipeg, Canada. Everywhere he went, and to all who would listen, he wailed about the sacrifice he was making in order to stay in shape.

He continues with his story that for a number of years he told his audiences that if you want to accomplish anything worthwhile you had to "pay the price." Then one day he was running on the grounds of Oregon State University. It was a beautiful, warm, spring day. He recalled how the ground was flowing effortlessly beneath his feet, he was breathing the fresh air and feeling about as good as one could wish to feel. Suddenly he knew he was having the time of his life. At the age of fifty he was in better shape than he was at twenty-five. He could run miles and miles without pain and drudgery. It was then, at that point, he had what could only be described as an epiphany. A deep and sudden knowing. The realization that hit him was this: You don't "pay the price" for good health – you enjoy the benefits of good health.

I cannot think of a more truthful or elegant statement.

You don't "pay the price" for good health – you enjoy the benefits of good health.

We have been so conditioned by our parents, teachers, media and "how-to" gurus that everything in life has a proportional cost/benefit ratio, the better the result the greater the cost.

You don't pay the price for success, you enjoy the benefits of success. You pay the price for failure. You don't pay the price for a good relationship, you enjoy the benefits of a good relationship. In essence, once you get the method down, it's the journey, and the enjoyment of that journey (which is your life) that brings all the benefits together.

On a personal level, when I first started to exercise regularly there were times during the first few weeks when I genuinely hated it. But it wasn't long before exercise turned into one of the most enjoyable parts of my day. I may often feel stiff and tired when I start, but before long I'm in the flow and my exercise time often becomes my meditation time as well.

I've never met a habitual jogger who doesn't crave the daily experience of running. Oh sure there are days when our "running friend" may not feel like lacing up the shoes, but watch this person if they experience an injury and they can't run for a couple of weeks. They're as anxious as a caged animal to get back to it. If they had any temporary delusions about paying the price those thoughts quickly vanish and they come to appreciate how fortunate they are when they can let their body loose and feel the boundless joys of physical activity and a healthy body.

CHAPTER NINETEEN
Do the *29 DAYS* courses guarantee I'll reach my goal in twenty-nine days?

If I want to lose thirty pounds in twenty-nine days will this actually happen?

29 DAYS is not about making outrageous promises it can't deliver. *Could* you lose thirty pounds in a month? Perhaps, but that isn't the objective of *29 DAYS*. The objective is to transform the way you think. The *29 DAYS* program will provide you with the necessary frame of mind to not only achieve your goal, but to maintain your new way of thinking ... effortlessly and permanently.

I hope you are convinced at this point that together, with your desire and the right method, (whether that's quitting smoking, building financial independence or becoming a great communicator etc.) you can accomplish any goal you desire.

Our goal in *29 DAYS* is to help you change your lifestyle not to help you go crazy bending yourself out of shape in a supreme effort toward losing weight, creating wealth, quitting smoking or any other goal you may desire. A successful *29 DAYS* course will change your deepest thoughts and habits in twenty-nine days so that you can enjoy a new lifestyle in an effortless and lasting manner.

Do we want you to achieve your desired habit? Obviously, and you will. But our ultimate goal is to see you change the way you think about your existing habit so that you end the struggle once and for all. As we said right from the very beginning, *you* will change, when the way you *think* changes. If you follow a *29 DAYS* course faithfully, in twenty-nine days you will have changed the way you think. Once changed, you will never be able to go back to your old way of thinking.

If you can't believe that something is possible, then you aren't going to have it. But if you can have the smallest belief that it might be possible, you are already on your way to creating it. You cannot create something if you cannot picture having it. Live out your dreams in your mind; picture and feel yourself getting what you want; hear the words you will say to others and what they will say to you when your dreams come true. You will learn to make your imaginings so real that they feel as if you have already achieved them rather than like wishful and distant fantasies.

> *29 DAYS* will help you to create a vision, to daydream and fantasize, and then focus each day on the simple, concrete steps you can take to reach your goal.

You will always take the path of least resistance. The path of least resistance is small, effortless, daily contributions towards your goal. In the case of wanting to lose weight, is that not easier than the daily resentment of being overweight, uncomfortable and unhealthy?

Logically, small simple steps *is* the path of least resistance. The biggest problem that we have in not choosing this path is that we want change to happen too quickly, and as a result we usually get nothing.

CHAPTER TWENTY
Above All Else, Enjoy the Journey!

This seemingly self-evident concept is unfortunately often overlooked by many of us. Ultimately it doesn't matter if we are the ideal weight, have a billion dollar bank account, and we enjoy perfect physical health, if we don't enjoy living our lives everything else is pretty much moot.

In *29 DAYS* we hope you take these courses in the spirit in which they are offered. Your goals to improve your life should do exactly that ... improve your life and make it truly more enjoyable.

News Flash! Each and Every One of Us Will Eventually Die.

It's true that most of us readily accept the fact that everyone, aside from ourselves of course, will die. I'm always amazed at how-to gurus, health nuts and prophets-of-doom who warn us that if we eat at fast-food joints, indulge in alcohol, eat red meat, ice cream and refined wheat, that we will surely die!

Let's take that argument to the next logical plateau – if we don't go to fast-food joints, if we cut out alcohol and abstain from eating red meat and ice cream, and instead subsist on broccoli and tofu – does that mean we're NOT going to die?!

Look, we all know that drastically cutting animal products, coffee, alcohol and everything else we enjoy is going to be better for our system, and quite frankly, if you can read a "what-you-should-do" book and incorporate that into your life you certainly don't need this program. If, on the other hand, you're like the majority of us, you're not about to embrace the life of a Himalayan monk because somebody suggests this is the path to a long life. Hey, how long do you want to live anyway if all you're allowed to consume is water, vegetables and tofu? With a menu like that we'd all be happily looking for a made-to-measure casket.

Okay, so let's get this straight, these *29 DAYS* courses are *not* about austerity and sacrifice.

I'm reminded of the story of Zig Ziglar who is being interviewed by his doctor after he's had a complete physical. The doctor suggested that if Ziglar were a building he'd be condemned. At this point Ziglar jumps in and says, "I suppose you're going to give me one of those diets that says you can't have this, and you can't have that, and be sure to stay away from this, and oh man, you certainly can't have that!"

To Ziglar's surprise his doctor responded with the most wonderful words a "condemned building" could imagine. "No," the doctor replied; "You can have anything you want!"

Just as Ziglar was about to acknowledge that that was one of the most beautiful replies he could have imagined the doctor continued with … "Now I'm going to tell you what you're going to want!"

Now of course this is a humorous little story, but the point is "bang on" and it's in complete alignment with the *29 DAYS* philosophy, which is NOT about depriving you of anything you want, but rather our goal is to change the way you think and ultimately what you *really do want.*

The better choices that you're really going to want aren't going to happen overnight. If you feel that *29 DAYS … to Your Perfect Weight,* or any of the other programs offered, is making you feel deprived, then you and the course are not in alignment. The goal is to change what you truly want in a healthy and lasting way. In a surprisingly short period of time many things that you truly want are going to be great choices that lead to your desired new behavior.

This is going to happen at a very subconscious level which is why it won't hurt and why it's going to last.

In his book *Creating Health*, Deepak Chopra writes:

> *If we want to create health, starting this moment, then we have to start channeling the unconscious mind through habit. In my experience, any approach to new habits should follow these guidelines: the habit should be acquired effortlessly over a period of time, it should be guided by positive thoughts, and it should be consciously repeated, but always in a good frame of mind, never forced in as the enemy of a bad habit. Cultivated in this way, new habits condition the whole mind-body system to create health and happiness automatically.*

While the actions you take to fulfill your goal may appear small, what you will accomplish is not. You will be building powerful habits and inner self-confidence that will transform you and make your life infinitely more enjoyable.

To commit your life to deeper relationships, financial security, peak physical health or a rewarding career is to enjoy the fruit that life begs us to take. These are simple yet powerful goals that will respond to powerful forces one gentle step at a time.

We invite you to join us in one of the *29 DAYS* courses and experience the power and thrill of permanent, positive, life-long change.

— <u>PART SIX</u> —

Let's Begin

CHAPTER TWENTY-ONE
How *29 DAYS* Courses Work

Once you have chosen your course from our list of available courses, you will need to register at our website at www.29daysto.com and fill in the required information.

Information Required:
- your email address
- starting date (choose the Monday you wish to begin)
- your time zone
- choose a picture from our picture library to visually chart your daily progress/or preferably send us your own inspirational picture

Daily Routine:

Morning:

29 DAYS and your online coach will be with you twice each day. In the morning we will prompt you to fulfill your daily step, read an inspiring message from your coach, or do a small simple task, or possibly just think about your goal for thirty seconds, or visualize something you will enjoy with the achievement of your goal, or ask your subconscious a question, etc. This daily morning message will come with a reply box that you will click when you have completed the day's step.

Evening:

When we have received your acknowledgement email that you have completed the day's step, we will send you 1/29th of your picture, as well as an inspirational message, story or some advice that you can consider, or turn over to your subconscious mind to consider, for the evening.

The daily routine will slowly build on each successive day until day twenty-nine. Every seven days we will prompt you to give yourself a reward for your patience and perseverance.

29 DAYS courses are based on four weeks, with each week having a target theme.

WEEK ONE: The first week is about commitment to your goal, and awareness of your present limiting habits and beliefs. Before you can neutralize the negative influences on your behavior, it is imperative that you become intimately aware of their existence. The first week you will focus on recognizing your habits, how and why you think the way you do, and to be absolutely certain that you are committed to change. This course is a four-part process with each week building on the previous week.

WEEK TWO: In week two you will begin to prepare yourself for action. You will begin to ask yourself simple but vital questions about how you might begin to make minor, but permanent changes to your behavior. These are changes that will almost seem too trivial to matter, but be assured, over time they will produce significant results.

WEEK THREE: By week three you will be wanting to take action. You will have spent the previous two weeks in decision and preparation. By day fifteen you will have a number of ideas and ways that you can tweak your lifestyle that will be relatively painless but will produce big results in a short period of time. And before you know it, it will be ...

WEEK FOUR: In week four you will be taking further action steps that will soon become habit. This week is really about driving home the concept that by maintaining the simple, yet painless changes you've made in week three, you are on the fast-track to a new life of effortless achievement and permanent results.

The daily changes you make in *29 DAYS* are small ...
the results are enormous

BOOK TWO

29 DAYS ... to your perfect weight

<u>HOW TO USE THE *29 DAYS* COURSES</u>

1. Be sure you have read *29 DAYS ... to a habit* you want! before you begin your course.

2. Register online to active your *29 DAYS* interactive coach.

3. Follow the daily program in the morning and evening. When you active your conscious and subconscious mind twice each day for twenty-nine days, you will create a powerful new way of thinking.

4. Do not skip ahead in the course. Follow each day and do the simple tasks as you receive them.

5. Enjoy! In just twenty-nine days you will have made a positive, and permanent change in your life.

Introduction

Welcome to *29 DAYS ... to your perfect weight.* Please be sure that you have read *29 DAYS ... to a habit you want!* before beginning this course. It's important that you understand the book's basic premise, which is: "We are the result of our thoughts; and that by changing our thoughts we can create or break our habits."

Thank you for agreeing to take this exciting journey. In the next four weeks you will be pleasantly surprised at the radical changes in your awareness and how you think about your weight, about eating and physical activity. These new thoughts will lead to a lifetime of living your perfect weight without regrets, anxiety or sacrifice.

There is one requirement on your part for the above statement to come true: You *must* really want to lose your excess weight. If you do, your thoughts and lifestyle will be radically different in just twenty-nine days and you'll never look back.

I've Been Where You Probably Are Right Now

Several years ago I was overweight and frustrated with myself. I think the biggest frustration was that there didn't seem to be any solutions to my dilemma. The insane world of diets and the latest weight-loss fads turned my stomach. I knew in my heart that if diets and fads were the only answer I would have to accept being overweight for the rest of my life. I couldn't see myself participating in that madness one more time. Then it happened. Using the principles of this course, I'm at a place I'm happy to be at ... for the rest of my life. This course will take you there too.

I must begin with a confession. If this confession sounds like a recording from an AA meeting forgive me but I have to say it: "My name is Michele and I've never been thin." Okay, there, I've said it.

Actually I've always had what I like to call an athlete's body type. I'm large boned. I have my mother's hips, gee thanks Mom. Muscle weighs more than fat. I was a competitive swimmer in my youth, hence the size of my thighs. These are some of the excuses I've used all of my life to justify my weight. Now, some of them may be relevant, like my hips for instance. They are what they are. Really and truly I will never have a body like Kate Moss. Come to think of it I don't want a body like Kate Moss. I just want to be a healthy weight ... for me.

When I was in my early forties I finally admitted to myself that my weight was getting out of control so I hired a physical trainer thinking this would help. I was willing to do anything she asked except for one small caveat; I refused to change my eating habits. From the beginning I made it very clear to her that I would work out four to five days a week, whatever was necessary, but under no circumstances was I going to change my eating habits. I just love food too much. I love to make it, eat it, and I thoroughly enjoy watching other people eat it.

I think about food from the moment I wake up in the morning until I go to bed at night. That doesn't mean that I necessarily eat food all day long, I just think about it all day long. By mid-morning I was thinking about what I was going to eat for lunch. By mid-afternoon I was mulling over what I was going to eat for dinner. I'm having company over on the weekend, hmm, I better think about that. What shall we eat?

So, my workout with my personal trainer began. My muscle tone became a little more defined. I grew a little stronger over time. I worked with her twice a week for almost two years. I would work out twice a week with her and twice a week on my own. After a good workout I would treat myself to something delicious. I earned it, I was working out! Hmm, I could justify that, unfortunately my body didn't seem to be buying into it since the one thing that didn't change was my weight. I did not lose one single pound!

So, what did I do? I did what any logical person would do ... I dropped my trainer. I didn't want to create more muscle, I wanted to shed the thirty pounds of excess weight. I felt frumpy, uncomfortable, and I had low self-esteem. I hated shopping for new clothes because I was embarrassed about the size I had to buy. I would look in the mirror with my clothes *on* and ask myself "What happened to me?" Don't even ask what I would say to myself while standing in front of the mirror naked!

Over a fifteen year period I had gained thirty plus pounds. That's equivalent to just two pounds a year, which doesn't really sound like much does it? Until you get on the scale one day and suddenly realize you are out of control. If I kept this up in a few years I'll be the size of my carport!

I dreaded the annual physicals. My doctor would raise her eyebrow and ever so gently mention that I had gained another five or ten pounds, and to think I went through the effort of not eating a crumb all day long before my afternoon appointment! When my doctor inquired about my daily habits I would naturally blush and tell her how much I worked out, how I ate healthy food and that I just couldn't understand why I wasn't able to lose any weight.

At some point I hit the wall. I decided to take action and do something about my weight once and for all. I finally realized that I actually did have to change my eating habits in order to lose weight. My challenge, and my deep inner fear was this: "Do I have to live the rest of my life feeling deprived? I love food, do I have to give up what I love? Do I have to live the rest of my life in a constant battle of willpower? Do I have to live the life of a deprived monk in order to lose weight? The moment I realized that answer was NO to each of those questions, my entire life changed.

I had an epiphany. I knew I had to change the way I thought about food, but it didn't mean feeling deprived. It didn't mean I had to give up one single thing. With this realization I got excited. Really excited. I strongly believe that the worst thing anyone can do when attempting to lose weight and improve one's health is to go on a diet. Your diet is just what you eat, and any improvement should be a step forward.

I had researched many weight-loss programs in the past, and I tried all the diets. By now I knew that I would never follow them, certainly not long term. To me these programs were about taking certain foods out of your life completely, and I knew I couldn't do that. Never have bread, pasta or chocolate again? Are you kidding me? As soon as you tell me I can't have something, my brain (that would be my amygdala) says I must have it, and have it in large quantities ... now!

Years earlier I had tried a program that stated: You can eat whatever you want but mind the size of the portions. I knew from experience that to lose weight, and keep it off, I had to:

- ✓ **Do it slowly over time.**
- ✓ **Train my brain.**
- ✓ **Forget trying to totally eliminate my favorite foods.**

So I begin, by writing down everything I ate, everyday, for the next week. I didn't change my eating habits. I wanted to know what my habits were. I found out two important things. I was a grazer. Yep, I unconsciously munched on something for most of the day. The second thing I discovered was that I had no concept of portion size. You mean a "platter" of pasta is not considered a single serving? Oh. Who would have thought?

Although I learned that it's a good idea to eat every two or three hours, it is *not* a good idea to eat an entire bag of chips, followed by a Snickers bar, and then round that off with a few handfuls of cashews.

This simple act of awareness really opened my eyes. I quickly began to consider the number of calories in a tablespoon of olive oil, a handful of salted nuts, a 14oz. steak. None of these things are necessarily good or bad yet it's important to be aware of "the facts, and nothing but the facts."

After I realized my habits, I started to deal with them one at a time ... slowly but surely.

Although I would wake up and think about food, I was never a breakfast eater. I knew it was "the most important meal of the day," however I usually didn't start my grazing until around nine. With my new awareness, I didn't change my eating schedule but I did change what I ate.

I still had my same lunch that I'd always brought to work, but instead of eating it all at noon, I would start into it around nine, and usually not finish it until three. This new pattern did a number of things:

- ✓ I wasn't randomly munching on whatever was in reach since I had already considered or screened what was going into my lunch when I made it.
- ✓ I never allowed myself to feel the sensation of hunger.
- ✓ It curbed my appetite before dinner.

Before becoming aware, I would get home from work and head straight for the refrigerator and grab a hunk of cheese or some deli meat to subside me. I didn't need to do that anymore because of my afternoon snack. I would keep a piece of fruit handy for my drive home as well. This simple act played a huge part in curbing my appetite.

Now, there was one other habit that I did notice while writing down everything I ate. I was an after dinner snacker. Okay, who isn't? Personally I'm a salt craver not a sweet craver. What I did to combat my salt craving was to eat a little healthier and a little less. Instead of potato chips, I'd munch on some homemade popcorn. Instead of tortilla chips, I would eat a few crackers. If I really "needed" chips, I would take some out of the bag and put them in a bowl.

Have you ever eaten chips out of the bag when you put your hand back into the bag and realize there is nothing left but the crumbs? It's happened to me more times than I care to admit. Another small change I made was my intake of water. I've always enjoyed water however I upped my intake. I had done quite a bit of research on water and its benefits, and as you'll see in this course, it's an incredibly powerful tool to health and weight loss.

About two or three months after I changed my daily habits, I "suddenly" had that indescribably delicious feeling, my clothes were becoming looser. I had more energy and when I stood on the scale (only once a week and on the same day) I was losing weight. At last! I had found the answer and it didn't hurt a bit!

After three or four months into my new lifestyle change, my best friend, whom I hadn't seen for a couple of months asked me the big question: "Have you lost weight?" I was so grateful to her. Someone actually noticed! This was really working! Hallelujah! I was ecstatic. I was so proud of myself.

Long story short, I lost thirty pounds over a period of nine months. That's an average of just over three pounds a month. Losing the weight is one thing, the real thrill, and daily joy, is that I've kept it off without the slightest discomfort and very little effort. I never feel deprived. What I feel is pride. It's hard to express how changing my thoughts and simple eating habits have affected my self-confidence and my self-esteem. Going on a diet is a very debilitating experience. You spend your entire day counting calories and thinking about what you can't have. That is not living. What joy and freedom it is to forget the diet fiasco and instead adopt a healthy lifestyle that will enhance your life both physically and emotionally.

I've keep the weight off because I changed my mind set. I changed the way I thought about food. Don't get me wrong, I still love to eat, and I do eat. I still love to cook, and I eat what I cook. All I did was make a few minor adjustments that over a short period of time literally transformed my life.

I want you to enjoy food, health and happiness the way I do. I want you to discover a new way of living that allows you to have everything you want and deprives you of nothing.
This course will interact with you twice a day making each day a step closer toward your goal – a lifetime of enjoying your perfect weight. It is a universal law of nature that we are the result of our thoughts and so for that reason, the first part of this course is designed for you to discover why you think the way you think about this area of your life. The cause of excess weight – barring a physical condition, is the result of the food we eat and the amount of physical activity we perform.

I will be your coach over the next twenty-nine days. I should add that although I'll be your coach, it's really *you* who will be discovering, and coaching your inner-self to permanent change and lasting results. I'll just be hanging around to offer a little guidance and moral support. As we said in the first section, the *Habits* book, you're going to learn how to do this all by yourself. Remember our motto from the Chinese Proverb:

> *Give a man a fish and you feed him for a day.*
> *Teach a man to fish and you feed him for a lifetime.*

Nothing of value can ever be created instantly. It doesn't matter if we are building a great business, learning to play an instrument, designing a building, getting an education, or even learning to ride a bicycle; each endeavor requires two things: 1. Patience/Perseverance and 2. Self-confidence.

You will need patience when it seems like you're moving too slowly and perseverance when it appears that no change is taking place. Without self-confidence we would never bother attempting anything because we would assume it would result in failure anyway. The greater your self-confidence, the greater the challenge you will attempt. If you commit to staying with us for the entire *29 DAYS ... to your perfect weight* course, it is an absolute promise that you will have all the patience, perseverance and self-confidence to achieve a lifetime of perfect weight.

Your program/course has been divided into four weeks, with each week building on the previous week. Each week you will be creating new neuron tracks/pathways, and embedding new ways of thinking and acting when it comes to food and physical activity.

Here's how the Four Week Program works...

Week One: Commitment and Awareness Week

In the first week you will establish two things: commitment and awareness. You have to be committed to losing your excess weight, or no power in the universe can cause this change. Through simple observation and awareness, you will begin to understand how you think about food and your overall health habits. You will simultaneously begin to build a strong foundation of commitment that will support you when the inevitable self-defeating excuses crop up that say, "This isn't working," or "This is taking too long."

Week Two: Preparation Week

Now that you have established awareness of your habits, and you know your inner-self is committed to achieving your goal, week two is designed to prepare you for action. You will begin to ask yourself simple but vital questions about how you might begin to make minor, but permanent changes to your behaviors. These are changes that will almost seem too trivial to matter, but over time they will produce significant results. By day ten or eleven, the daily reminders, your visualization and simple affirmations will already be forming powerful new neuron tracks. These new thought patterns will begin to produce deep-seated lifelong changes. Your self-confidence and personal power will begin to show signs of life!

Week Three: Taking Action

By now you'll be wanting to take action, and that is precisely the time to take it! You will have spent the previous two weeks in awareness, decision and preparation. By day fifteen you will have a number of ideas and ways that you can tweak your lifestyle that will be painless but will simultaneously produce big results in a short period of time.

Week Four: Staying the Course

Beginning in week four you will be taking action steps that will be life transforming. This week is really about driving home the concept that by maintaining the simple, yet painless changes you made in week three, you are on track to a new life of effortlessly losing the rest of your excess weight, and most importantly to keeping it off forever. This is the week that you alter your thinking from a goal to a life-long commitment. Your goal may still be to lose twenty, thirty, forty or more extra pounds, but by now you will be making a commitment and a deep-seated promise to live a life with new thought patterns and new awareness. In fact, after you have taken the entire *29 DAYS* course, it will no longer be possible for you to return to your old eating habits and thought patterns.

Enough talk already. Let's get started!

— <u>WEEK ONE</u> —

COMMITMENT AND AWARENESS

DAY ONE
Awareness Is Vital
To Fundamental Change

DAY ONE - A.M.

Welcome to *29 DAYS ... to your perfect weight.*

STEP 1– For today, try to be aware of everything you eat and drink and that means everything. Even the little nibbles that you think don't count... but do.

Today's goal is to simply begin to create awareness. Try to notice when you eat. When are you hungry? Are you ever hungry? When do you think about food? Is it often? What do you think about it? What kind of food do you think about? What type of eating do you think about - snacks, meals? Do you tend to eat to refuel? For entertainment? For emotional fulfillment?

So today's step is to simply try and be aware and to notice your thoughts and habits. That's it. Be honest with yourself. Please be as diligent as you can ... try to catch absolutely everything.

Note: Do not attempt to change your behavior or eating patterns at this time. This first week is about creating awareness. Simple, basic awareness is vital to achieving permanent results.

> AWARENESS IS VITAL TO FUNDAMENTAL CHANGE

JOURNAL ENTRY

For the rest of today please try to be aware of the following questions:

How often did I eat today and at what times? _half a dozen times/whenever_

Was I ever hungry today and if so, when was it? _mid-morning_

What, if anything, prompted me to think about eating? _taste_

What time of the day do I crave a snack? _whenever_

What kind of food do I like to snack on? _diet/nutritional food_

Did I eat out of habit or physical hunger? _habit / once a day hunger_

Did I eat or drink for entertainment? _yes_

Did I eat for emotional fulfillment? _____

Did I catch myself eating without even being aware? _no_

How much water did I drink today? _I hate water_

DAY ONE – P.M. MESSAGE

I hope you had a great day.

Did You Know?

Am I full yet? The question may take longer to answer than you may think. It takes fifteen minutes or more for the message that we're full to get from our stomachs to our brains.

Think back to the beginning of the day and fill in your Food and Drink Log on the facing page. It's especially important to try and note what caused you to eat and drink. Was it thirst, hunger, emotions, habit, boredom, location, duty? Whatever it is try to determine the underlying cause.

For the rest of Awareness week you're going to be asked to fill out your daily food

FOOD AND DRINK CONSUMPTION - DAY ONE

TIMES I ATE	WHAT I ATE	WHAT CAUSED ME TO EAT
Early Morning	Hummus Caches	Hunger/Doubt of all others
Mid-Morning	Shake	Frying to forget food
Lunch		
Afternoon		
Before Dinner		
Dinner		
After Dinner		
Late Evening		

TIMES I DRANK	WHAT I DRANK	WHAT CAUSED ME TO DRINK
Morning	Pop (Cherry)	Taste / Thirst
Mid Morning	" "	"
Lunch		
Afternoon		
Dinner		
Evening		

Remember: Do not try and change your habits and behaviors at this time. Just note and record your daily eating and drinking activity. First comes understanding, then comes change.

Week One: Commitment and Awareness ~ 125

and drink log. There's nothing for you to change at this point, awareness is all that matters.

Awareness Is Vital To Fundamental Change

Please consider the following questions:

Was I ever hungry today and if so, when was it? _Not hungry_

What, if anything, prompted me to think about eating? _I'd not cheated_

What time of the day do I crave a snack? _Am_

What kind of food do I like to snack on? _Lettce / cherries / nuts_

feel about losi wt

_____

_____

Do I eat out of habit or physical hunger? _habit_

Did I eat or drink for entertainment? _eat_

Did I eat for emotional fulfillment? _(yes)_

Did I catch myself eating without even being aware? _no_

Is there anything I discovered today about my eating, or thoughts about eating, that surprised me? _I'm afraid of losy wt._

Nothing tastes as good as being thin feels.
~Author Unknown

See you tomorrow.

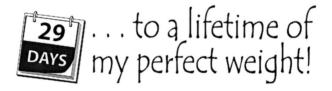

29 DAYS . . . to a lifetime of my perfect weight!

DAY TWO
Awareness Is Vital
To Fundamental Change

DAY TWO – A.M.

Welcome back, we're on our way. Today's step is a continuation of step one. Yesterday you began to notice and track some of your habitual thoughts about food and drink, when you may eat and drink and why. It will take a few days to really notice a pattern. Remember, awareness is the first crucial step toward changing your habitual thoughts.

STEP 2 - Today's goal is to generate greater awareness of your eating and drinking habits and patterns.

Why do you want to lose weight? What will losing weight do for you? How will it make you feel? How will losing weight enhance your life? This is a very vital step.

Try to be aware of the following: Try to notice when you eat. When are you hungry? Are you ever hungry? When do you think about food? Is it often? What do you think about it? What kind of food do you think about? Is there something that triggers a desire for food? Does it produce a particular feeling? Remember to write everything down, even the little things.

As you know, our lives are the results of our thoughts, so try to notice what thoughts trigger what response. For the rest of today, please try to be aware of everything you eat and drink. Jot down your thoughts, feelings and discoveries.

JOURNAL ENTRY

Awareness Is Vital To Fundamental Change

Why do I want to lose weight? _Attractive/Healthy; but the attraction scares me_

What will losing weight do for me? _I won't have so many thoughts swimming thru my head, I'll fit in, I'll find her, maybe._

How will I feel if I could live my life at my desired weight? _less worried about death_

In what ways will my life be enhanced if I was to become my perfect weight? _____

DAY TWO – P.M. MESSAGE

Give yourself a pat on the back for being here and for being aware of everything you ate and drank today.

The second day of a diet is always easier than the first. By the second day, you're off it.
~ Jackie Gleason

Thank goodness you're <u>not</u> on a diet!

FOOD AND DRINK CONSUMPTION - DAY TWO

TIMES I ATE	WHAT I ATE	WHAT CAUSED ME TO EAT
Early Morning		
Mid-Morning	Yogurt ½Baren Cereal	I dee of it/Taste
Lunch	Almonds	
Afternoon		
Before Dinner		
Dinner		
After Dinner		
Late Evening		
TIMES I DRANK	WHAT I DRANK	WHAT CAUSED ME TO DRINK
Morning		
Mid Morning		
Lunch		
Afternoon		
Dinner		
Evening		

Remember: Do not try and change your habits and behaviors at this time. Just note and record your daily eating and drinking activity. First comes understanding, then comes change.

The Power of Visualization

There are two times of the day that your subconscious mind is most receptive – when you first wake up and when you are just about to fall asleep. When you wake up try and picture how you would like to look. Can you picture yourself in a great pair of jeans, or pulling your belt in by an extra couple of notches? Imagine yourself at a family reunion and hear people complimenting how good you look. Imagine going to a store and purchasing clothes that are a couple of sizes smaller than what you presently wear. How about seeing yourself playing tennis, or walking along the beach looking just the way you'd like to look. Even doing so for ten seconds will have a powerful effect after a short period of time.

Since this is the last message for today, try to remember visualizing the way you would like to see yourself just as you are about to drift off to sleep. This will begin to set up active and magnetic forces unlike anything you can believe. Remember, the last thing you think of before you go to sleep is what your subconscious mind has to work with all night long. Whatever your subconscious mind consistently has to work with, you will consistently move toward.

Since you're always thinking about something just before you go to sleep, you might just as well train yourself to think of something you desire!

Whatever the mind of man can conceive and believe, it can achieve.
~ Napoleon Hill

See you tomorrow!

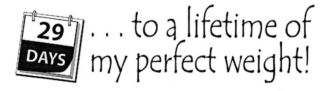

DAY THREE
Awareness Is Vital
To Fundamental Change

DAY THREE – A.M.

Welcome to day three. As you can well imagine, it takes a period of time to notice if we follow certain habits or patterns. For today try to notice any recurring patterns you have toward *what* and *when* you eat and drink. Does your mood affect your eating habits? Is it the time of day? Are you really hungry when you eat? How often do you eat? Do you eat when you're bored? Are the portions you eat large? Could they be slightly smaller? Could you substitute the foods you eat for a different type of food or perhaps a different activity?

STEP 3 – Since it's day three and you're still here, you're obviously serious about losing your excess weight. Each of us have our reasons, and discovering your reasons is a vital step. Please be sure you have *written down* your reasons for wanting to lose weight. You don't have to do this in the next five minutes or even five hours, but *do* jot down as many reasons as you can think of. By day's end you may have several reasons and by tomorrow you may have thought of a few more. This is a very important step so please be sure to write down as many benefits as you can think of for wanting to lose your excess weight. Also, please continue to notice and be aware of everything you eat and drink.

We have talked about the power of visualization and creating mental pictures. Here is a very powerful way to help you create a mental image of the way you wish to look. Find a picture in a magazine or photo album of a person (perhaps even yourself at your ideal weight) who has the kind of body you would like to have. Cut off the head and put a picture of your face there instead. Put this picture in your snack drawer or refrigerator. If you don't want anyone to see it, then put it in your

> *Please, please do this simple exercise, you will find it extremely powerful.*

desk drawer or car, but put it somewhere where you will see it several times each day. Make a few copies and put them in several areas where you will see them throughout your day. Every time you see yourself with the body you desire, your subconscious mind will be making powerful neuron connections that will propel you toward your goal.

JOURNAL ENTRY

Awareness Is Vital To Fundamental Change

Does my mood affect my eating habits? _____

_____

Do I automatically eat because it's a certain time of day? _____

_____

What are my food triggers? Watching television? Starting up my computer? Reading a book?

_____

_____

Do I tend to eat a lot at once or nibble? _____

Is there anything I discovered today about my eating, or thoughts about eating, that
   surprised me? _____

_____

If I can find a good enough reason to change, I'll change!

In what ways will my life be enhanced when I become my perfect weight?_____

_____

FOOD AND DRINK CONSUMPTION - DAY THREE

TIMES I ATE	WHAT I ATE	WHAT CAUSED ME TO EAT
Early Morning		
Mid-Morning		
Lunch		
Afternoon		
Before Dinner		
Dinner		
After Dinner		
Late Evening		
TIMES I DRANK	**WHAT I DRANK**	**WHAT CAUSED ME TO DRINK**
Morning		
Mid Morning		
Lunch		
Afternoon		
Dinner		
Evening		

Remember: Do not try and change your habits and behaviors at this time. Just note and record your daily eating and drinking activity. First comes understanding, then comes change.

DAY THREE – P.M. MESSAGE

Congratulations, you've completed three full days!

When you go to bed this evening, and just before you go to sleep, repeat to yourself:

"I am my perfect weight and healthy."

Say this as you visualize yourself looking just like you do in the picture you cut out today.

Remember, the last thing you think of before you go to sleep is what your subconscious mind has to work with all night long.

See you tomorrow!

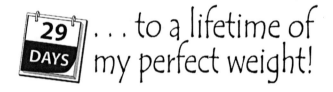

... to a lifetime of my perfect weight!

DAY FOUR
Awareness Is Vital
To Fundamental Change

DAY FOUR - A.M.

Welcome to day four. Congratulations for getting this far. Your inner-self-doubts have been working outside your conscious awareness, fighting to stop any change to your lifestyle. Fortunately, you have patience and perseverance and so, here you are!

By now you must be noticing your eating habits and traits. Please jot some of them down in your journal for future reference. Write down anything that you think relates to either an eating habit or a reactive response to your "automatic" thoughts.

Let's consider the following:

Regardless of your age, genetics, metabolism or exercise program, your ability to lose weight will ultimately boil down to pure physics – burn more than you consume. Losing excess weight breaks down as follows: If you desire to lose one pound per week, you will need to burn 3,500* more calories than you consume. That amounts to 500 calories per day. This breaks down to eliminating one can of regular soda and a small bag of potato chips each day. This 500 calorie reduction could be the elimination of a daily donut and fast-food take out three times a week. There is nothing for you to try and eliminate at this point, this is merely "food" for thought.

> ** Please note: The above explanation is based on the assumption that you are holding steady on your excess weight. In other words, you were x pounds overweight last year and you're still x pounds overweight right now. If, you are steadily gaining weight, you will need to lose more than 500 calories each day for positive weight reduction.*

STEP 4 - Whatever it is that you are eating daily, think about what it might be that is causing you to either gain weight, or not take it off. We are only talking about reducing 500 calories each day in order for you to lose one pound each week. If you were to eliminate that daily, 500 calorie consumption (whatever that might be) and perhaps enjoy that food or drink once a week instead, how much difference in weight would that make in just six months? Would you believe that would add up to a loss of more than twenty pounds without any physical exertion whatsoever! Losing that amount of weight each week is within healthy guidelines for permanent weight loss.

So here is some further food-for-thought. There is nothing for you to do at this stage, except just consider the above information. Do you think that eliminating 500 calories a day is within the realm of possibility for you?

Although there is no shortage of testimonials of people losing ten pounds in ten days, or thirty pounds in a month, this is neither a healthy nor desirable outcome. Sudden weight reduction caused by artificial changes to our eating habits, or starvation as a result of low-calorie diets, will inevitably lead to further problems. Rapid weight loss doesn't allow for healthy or sustainable habits. Although our physical weight may have changed, our mental approach to food and eating hasn't. When one's willpower runs out, and it will, dieters inevitably regain all the lost weight.

The human body is not designed to shed weight, it's designed to survive! If you drastically reduce your calorie-intake, your brain takes active steps to slow down your metabolism to conserve calories. Eating too few calories robs you of energy and often leads to uncontrollable food cravings.

Too rapid weight loss results in loss of water and muscle ... both of which are vital to a healthy body. In addition to the physical cost, visually the skin does not have time to shrink to the new body shape resulting in leaving one looking like a shar pei puppy. The crash dieter's next pursuit may be skin surgery!

JOURNAL ENTRY

Awareness Is Vital To Fundamental Change

What pattern have I noticed about my eating habits? _____

_____

_____

What, if anything, happens in my daily life that triggers a desire to eat?_____

_____

_____

If I can find a good enough reason to change, I'll change!

I know that there isn't any action to take today other than to continue to be aware of my

eating habits. By being aware, however, have I noticed some small step that I might

take in the future that would cause me to either consume less calories or burn some

extra calories? _____

_____

_____

_____

A small step that might cause me to consume less calories is: _____

_____

A small step that might cause me to burn a few extra calories is: _____

_____

"Patience and perseverance have a magical effect before which
difficulties disappear and obstacles vanish."
~ John Quincy Adams

FOOD AND DRINK CONSUMPTION - DAY FOUR

TIMES I ATE	WHAT I ATE	WHAT CAUSED ME TO EAT
Early Morning		
Mid-Morning		
Lunch		
Afternoon		
Before Dinner		
Dinner		
After Dinner		
Late Evening		
TIMES I DRANK	WHAT I DRANK	WHAT CAUSED ME TO DRINK
Morning		
Mid Morning		
Lunch		
Afternoon		
Dinner		
Evening		

Remember: Do not try and change your habits and behaviors at this time. Just note and record your daily eating and drinking activity. First comes understanding, then comes change.

DAY FOUR – P.M. MESSAGE

Congratulations on another successful day. If you promise to stay the course, we promise that you will easily reach your goal of Your Perfect Weight.

When you go to bed this evening, and just before you go to sleep, repeat to yourself:

"I am my perfect weight and healthy."

Say this as you visualize yourself looking just like you do in the picture you cut out yesterday. When you visualize, picture yourself at your ideal weight and begin to own that picture of yourself. You can visualize exactly the way you want your body to look knowing that you're on a path of achievement and that you cannot fail. You are programming your future because your mind will move in that direction automatically.

Remember, the last thing you think of before you go to sleep is what your subconscious mind has to work with all night long.

A "successful life" is nothing more than a sum total of many "successful years."
A successful year is the compilation of a dozen successful months.
A successful month is the result of four successful weeks,
which in turn, is seven successful days.
If you can make today a successful day,
then a wonderfully successful life will be yours one day at a time.

See you tomorrow.

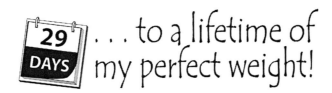 . . . to a lifetime of my perfect weight!

DAY FIVE
Awareness Is Vital
To Fundamental Change

DAY FIVE - A.M.

Hey, welcome back. We're on day five and you're still hanging in. Congratulations!

By now you're beginning to recognize some strong habits. These habits probably begin with a thought and finish with an action – perhaps the thought of food pops into your head and the natural result may very well be eating. Being aware of your thoughts and recognizing patterns is a huge weapon toward defeating those inner-doubts and subsequently achieving your goals.

As we said earlier, before a goal can realistically be accomplished there has to be a commitment. This commitment is crucial to carry you over, under, around and through the self-defeating beliefs that your inner-self will send your way.

Since this *first week* is about commitment and awareness, you will also need to be aware of every trick your inner-self (amygdala) has in store so that you won't be caught unaware.

You have decided that you want to become your *Perfect Weight*. Wonderful. Ask yourself, are there any negative consequences to losing weight?

You're first reaction might be "What, are you kidding? How could there be any negatives about losing my excess weight? Think deeper. If you lost 30, 40, 50 or 100 pounds, would that affect your spouse? Maybe positively. Maybe negatively. What if your spouse is also 30, 40, 50 or 100 pounds overweight? Would he or she feel negatively toward the new you? Would it mean having to buy a whole new wardrobe? We're not suggesting that there is anything wrong with buying a whole new wardrobe or that you should *not* lose weight because your spouse may have a streak of jealousy or that your spouse simply wants things to remain the same. We are just cautioning you that you need to be mindful of these potential issues before you set your goal.

By being aware of these issues now, you will be prepared when those self-defeating thoughts pop up ... and they will. That's your amygdala. Let it know who's in control. When the inevitable negative thoughts arrive you can readily dismiss them as "been there, done that."

Remember: The more important your goal is to you, the more your inner-self will try to keep you from going after it. Your inner-self sees an important goal as frightening, difficult and a potential for failure. It would prefer that you not attempt anything new so that there's no risk of failure!

Note: One of the amygdala's self-doubt tricks will be to instill the fear of having to live a life of austerity. It will have you falsely imagine having to subsist on nothing but raw vegetables, tofu and bran.

As we've pointed out many times, enjoying a life at your perfect weight is not an all-or-nothing proposition. In fact your amygdala will try to tell you that giving up a small portion here and there will take too long, or it won't be effective. Don't you believe it! You're going to love your new eating habits. You'll feel in control, proud, healthy, and confident. You will *not* feel deprived. That is why you will be able to change your thoughts, your desires and enjoy a life-time of being your perfect weight. Stay with us. This can be fun.

STEP 5 - Please take a few moments and consider what possible tricks your inner-self (amygdala) might drag out of the recesses of your mind when you might be most susceptible to self-doubt in a week or two from now. Jot them down, so that if/when they come, you can confidently dismiss them for the self-defeating, double-crossing tactics that they are.

JOURNAL ENTRY

Awareness Is Vital To Fundamental Change

Are there any possible negative consequences to becoming my perfect weight? _____

_____

_____

When I become my perfect weight will it effect any of my relationships in a negative way?

_____

_____

Will I have to purchase a new wardrobe? If so, is it something I look forward to doing or would it be a financial strain? _____

_____

If a new wardrobe could be a financial issue, might I be able to cut back on my food or social-drink budget when I begin to lose weight so that the savings would offset the cost of some new clothes? _____

Please write this statement out and give it a moment of consideration as you do.

> I have tried to lose weight in the past but I was never able to be successful for the long term. I remember losing weight but then I would get these thoughts that would pop into my head and urge me to forget weight loss and binge instead. These thoughts came from my amygdala, which hates to see change.

_____

_____

_____

_____

_____

In the past, some of my amygdala's excuses to forget weight loss and eat whatever and whenever I want were: _____

_____

_____

FOOD AND DRINK CONSUMPTION - DAY FIVE

TIMES I ATE	WHAT I ATE	WHAT CAUSED ME TO EAT
Early Morning		
Mid-Morning		
Lunch		
Afternoon		
Before Dinner		
Dinner		
After Dinner		
Late Evening		

TIMES I DRANK	WHAT I DRANK	WHAT CAUSED ME TO DRINK
Morning		
Mid Morning		
Lunch		
Afternoon		
Dinner		
Evening		

Remember: Do not try and change your habits and behaviors at this time. Just note and record your daily eating and drinking activity. First comes understanding, then comes change.

DAY FIVE – P.M. MESSAGE

Congratulations on sticking with the program and for jotting down your positive and negative thoughts about attaining your goal.

Right about here you might be thinking that this course isn't moving very fast. After all, you're five days into it and you haven't been asked to lose an ounce. What gives?

Just hang in there. Continue to follow the program and you will see the results. In some ways twenty-nine days doesn't seem like a long time, but in other ways it may seem like an eternity. Keep doing the daily steps and at the end you will look back at the twenty-nine day span from a very different perspective. You will have drastically changed how you think ... permanently. You're going to cover a lot of ground both physically and mentally. Please remember, slow gentle effortless steps doesn't mean that your progress will mirror that. Slow, gentle effortless steps will produce enormous results. Patience and perseverance is the key. Patience and perseverance.

It won't be long before you can begin to <u>see</u> the achievement of your goal.

> *"You've got to say, I think that if I keep working at this and want it badly enough I can have it. It's called perseverance."*
> *~ Lee Iacocca*

See you tomorrow.

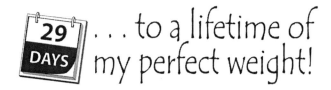

DAY SIX
Awareness Is Vital
To Fundamental Change

DAY SIX - A.M.

Welcome back, you're doing great!

Yesterday you jotted down some possible arguments your inner-self may be stockpiling in an attempt to derail you at a later date. These written steps are very important to build two things:

1. a solid mental foundation, and
2. creating new neuron tracks that will lead you to the enjoyment of a lifetime of being your healthy weight.

As you can well imagine, it's rather impossible to arrive at a destination if we don't have one.

Without a destination or goal, we're simply wandering about – much like Alice in Lewis Carroll's *Alice in Wonderland* when, not sure of where she wanted to go, she asked the Cheshire Cat for directions.

> *"Cheshire-Puss," she began, rather timidly ... "would you tell me, please, which way I ought to go from here?"*
>
> *"That depends a good deal on where you want to get to," said the Cat.*
>
> *"I don't much care where—," said Alice.*
>
> *"Then it doesn't matter which way you go," said the Cat.*

Alice's statement about not caring where she wanted to go, and the cat's response that it didn't matter then which way she went, pretty much sums up "a life without a goal." But you're different. You're going to set and achieve a goal, and in order to set it properly we want to give you a bit of direction and guidance.

On day eight you will write out two goals. The first goal will be what you wish to accomplish by the end of this course. The second goal will be your lifetime goal, or better still, a lifestyle that you wish to live by.

Goals and affirmations have a magical way of unlocking your subconscious mind, which will begin to release ideas and energy for your goal attainment. Clearly written and well thought out goals and affirmations will increase your self-confidence and enhance your levels of motivation.

By simply deciding exactly what you want to achieve, you will begin to move unerringly toward your goal, and your goal will start to move unerringly toward you.

There are two ways to think about goals. You can write a goal for your conscious mind and you can also create a goal for your subconscious mind. There is a difference.

Conscious Mind: Goals

Your conscious mind thinks in terms of time: past, present and future. If your goal is to lose thirty pounds then a clearly written, conscious goal might be written like this:

I weigh 155 pounds on x date.

This is a goal that is written in a positive tense with a specific time.

Subconscious Mind: Goals

Your subconscious mind has no concept of time. It only functions in the present. Therefore when you communicate with your subconscious mind you will do so in the form of an affirmation. A goal for your conscious mind written as: "I weigh 155 pounds on x date," would become an affirmation to your subconscious mind that you would repeat as, "I weigh 155 pounds." The only difference is that you don't put a date on it. You relay this desire to your subconscious mind and it will find the shortest route to your goal.

You put the date on it for your conscious mind so that it becomes a believable goal for you. This aligns the believability your conscious mind needs to the positive, emotional feeling that fuels your subconscious mind.

As noted earlier, our subconscious mind is our success tool, and unfortunately we were never taught how to use it effectively. If you wish to eliminate a bad habit it is imperative to write your goal in a positive/positive way.

Your goals for *A Lifetime of Your Perfect Weight* must have the following characteristics:

Written goals for your Conscious Mind

1. It must be something that you really want – since you're still with the course, this one can definitely be checked off.
2. It must be clear, measureable and specific with a definite date on it. For example: "On x date I weigh 155 pounds.

Written Goals/Affirmations for Your Subconscious Mind

1. Your affirmation goals must be positive because your subconscious mind cannot process a negative command. It is only receptive to a positive, present tense statement. In this case, you wouldn't write, "I want to lose a few pounds," or even "I want to lose fifteen pounds."

2. When communicating with your subconscious mind, you should always state and write your goals in a positive, present and personal way. So, by positive, we mean that you don't write what you don't want. Example: *I don't want to be overweight*, or *I don't want to overeat*. Positive means, "I am the perfect weight," or "I eat just the right amount." These are positive statements. Present statements mean that your goal is written in the present tense. Again you wouldn't write: "I will lose 15 pounds," but rather, "I weigh x number of pounds."

Writing, "I will become ..." keeps it in the future and "I want ..." keeps you longing and never having. All *wanting* affirms the *not having* - to your subconscious mind.

Finally your goal must be both measurable and quantifiable. To meet this requirement you merely need to fill in some specifics. So instead of saying "I want to lose weight," you would say the specific amount and the time period in which it will happen.

3. It must be believable and achievable. People will often say: "Hey, I thought you said that anybody can achieve anything that 'the mind can conceive

and believe'?" That's true to a point. If for example you say; "I will live forever," your subconscious mind won't buy into it which means you're wasting your time.

Shaquille O'Neal is a 7' 1'', 325-pound world-famous basketball player who happens to have many interests. One of his interests is law enforcement. Now if Shaq decided he wants to become an undercover cop when he retires from basketball, or if he wants to become a thoroughbred racehorse jockey, it doesn't matter how badly he wants it, it's not happening! We have to make sure that what we're setting our hearts on is within the accepted realms of what our conscious and subconscious mind will buy into. If our subconscious mind won't buy into it, it won't offer the required support.

STEP 6 – You won't be asked to write out your goals today. The above information is being given to you a couple of days early because it will give your conscious and subconscious some time to mull things over.

There is nothing further for you to do today except continue to notice any additional thoughts or patterns you have about eating and their subsequent reactions. Please remember to visualize yourself at your ideal weight for a moment or two whenever you can. Make sure you're looking at the picture you cut out showing your face on your ideal body.

JOURNAL ENTRY

Awareness Is Vital To Fundamental Change

Affirmations are similar in outcome to cutting a path through scrub brush. The more you walk the same path, the easier it becomes. Frequently citing an affirmation creates an indelible groove in your subconscious mind. The more you recite or think about a positive affirmation, the quicker your subconscious will work toward its attainment.

I like this affirmation because I can recite it easily, I believe it in my heart and I know it will soon be mine:

Examples: "Losing body fat is easy and effortless for me."
"Nothing tastes as good as being thin feels."
"My body is getting slimmer every day."

If I can find a good enough reason to change, I'll change!

Possible ideas for my weight loss goals: _____

_____

_____

It would be far easier to lose weight permanently
if replacement parts weren't so handy in the refrigerator.
~ Hugh Allen

DAY SIX – P.M. MESSAGE

You can be sure that your subconscious mind is already considering your goals – the short-term goal for this course as well as the longer one – a lifestyle goal.

When you go to bed this evening, and just before you go to sleep, begin applying the powerful tool of affirmations. Repeat to yourself: "I am my perfect weight and healthy." Say this a number of times as you visualize yourself looking just like you do in the picture you cut out in STEP 3.

See and feel how proud you'll be when you reach your goal.

You're almost one quarter of the way there! You're doing great, keep on going!

I do not think there is any other quality so essential to success of any kind,
as the quality of perseverance. It overcomes almost everything in nature.
~ John D. Rockefeller ~

Remember whatever you focus on is what the subconscious believes you want.

See you tomorrow!

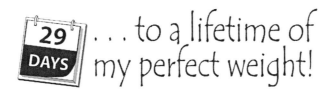

FOOD AND DRINK CONSUMPTION - DAY SIX

TIMES I ATE	WHAT I ATE	WHAT CAUSED ME TO EAT
Early Morning		
Mid-Morning		
Lunch		
Afternoon		
Before Dinner		
Dinner		
After Dinner		
Late Evening		
TIMES I DRANK	WHAT I DRANK	WHAT CAUSED ME TO DRINK
Morning		
Mid Morning		
Lunch		
Afternoon		
Dinner		
Evening		

Remember: Do not try and change your habits and behaviors at this time. Just note and record your daily eating and drinking activity. First comes understanding, then comes change.

DAY SEVEN
Awareness Is Vital
To Fundamental Change

DAY SEVEN - A.M.

Guess what? You're twenty-five percent of the way there and today you've earned a reward! It's important to keep this reward *small*. Small rewards have a magical way of stimulating your internal motivation.

If you're feeling any doubt or resistance to granting yourself a reward for your efforts thus far … perish the thought, it's just your inner-self marshalling its negative forces. Your inner-voice might suggest, "You don't deserve a reward for something you should be doing anyway," or "I don't feel I should give myself a reward, I haven't done anything yet," or "It doesn't feel right" and so on.

You *have* earned a reward. You've completed six days of a course that you didn't have to do, so there's no earthly reason that you shouldn't reward yourself. Research shows that tangible rewards provide psychological motivation. Rewards are the easiest, most effective psychological motivators known.

When thinking of a reward, think small. Small rewards are a form of recognition rather than becoming an end in themselves.

Your reward should have the following two qualities:
✓ **It should be appropriate to your goal.**
✓ **It should be free or inexpensive.**

What's an Appropriate Reward?

One that supports your goal. If your goal was to quit drinking alcohol, then clearly a celebration reward with a bottle of champagne would be somewhat counter-productive. In your case, let's not associate a reward with any food or drink. Let's think of some other small rewards that would not detract from your goal.

What Reward Could You Give Yourself that Would be Free or Inexpensive?

Inexpensive is certainly a relative term. After all, if you're an overweight Saudi Sheik taking this course you may consider a small reward as going for an afternoon cruise on your yacht! However, for the rest of us "poor schleps," here are a few suggestions: go see a movie, rent a movie, buy a paperback, call a friend, enjoy some TV time, listen to a great piece of music, go for a walk, buy a magazine, etc. Think of something that you may not normally do and "DO IT!" It's important to do something you really enjoy doing.

STEP 7 – Think of a reward and make sure you enjoy it … today! Enjoy!

> **Possible Ideas for a Reward:**
> • Give yourself a manicure
> • Read a book
> • Go for a walk
> • Watch a movie or TV
> • Buy a Magazine
> • Play a round of golf or a game of tennis

If I can find a good enough reason to change, I'll change!

DAY SEVEN – P.M. MESSAGE

We hope you had a great day and that you took the time to enjoy your reward.

Awareness Is Vital To Fundamental Change

For my reward I gave myself:_____

The first week is complete.

FOOD AND DRINK CONSUMPTION - DAY SEVEN

TIMES I ATE	WHAT I ATE	WHAT CAUSED ME TO EAT
Early Morning		
Mid-Morning		
Lunch		
Afternoon		
Before Dinner		
Dinner		
After Dinner		
Late Evening		

TIMES I DRANK	WHAT I DRANK	WHAT CAUSED ME TO DRINK
Morning		
Mid Morning		
Lunch		
Afternoon		
Dinner		
Evening		

Remember: Do not try and change your habits and behaviors at this time. Just note and record your daily eating and drinking activity. First comes understanding, then comes change.

Week One was all about awareness and commitment. I know I'm committed to losing my excess weight.

By directing my attention and awareness toward my daily eating habits I learned some interesting things about myself. I learned: _____

_____

_____

_____

_____

_____

_____

For the past seven days you have been recording your daily intake of food and drink. By now you will have a clear picture of your eating and drinking habits and behaviors. The upcoming week will begin a new focus and a new thought process. You will begin to build your resolve and continue to reinforce your commitment to achieving your perfect weight and health. Week two is going to get you mentally prepared for effortless action in week three.

You have successfully finished twenty-five percent of the course. That's great. You really did earn your reward you know.

See you tomorrow.

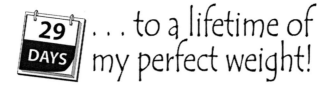

— <u>WEEK TWO</u> —

PREPARATION FOR ACTION

DAY EIGHT
I'm the best reason in the world to change ... so I'll change!

DAY EIGHT - A.M.

Welcome to Week Two. In the first week you accomplished two very important things toward building a foundation toward a lifetime of your *perfect weight*. You established awareness of your habits, and you confirmed your commitment to enjoying a lifetime of being your *perfect weight*.

Week two is PREPARATION WEEK. This is the week that will get you fully prepared for action in week three. You will begin this week by asking yourself simple but vital questions about how you might begin to make minor, but permanent changes to your eating habits and behaviors.

Remember, we want small changes. They may even seem too trivial to matter, but over time they will produce significant results. The daily reminders, your visualizations, affirmations and simple rewards are now forming powerful new neuron tracks. These new thought patterns are beginning to produce deep-seated change.

Written goals and affirmations have a magical way of unlocking your subconscious mind which will begin to release ideas and energy for your goal attainment. Clearly written and well thought out goals will increase your self-confidence and enhance your levels of motivation. By simply deciding exactly what you want, you will begin to move unerringly toward your goal, and your goal will start to move unerringly toward you.

Recap to Setting Your Goals

Conscious Mind: Goals

Your conscious mind thinks in terms of time: past, present and future. If your goal is to lose thirty pound then a clearly written, conscious goal might be written like this: I weigh 155 pounds on x date. This is a goal that is written in a positive tense with a specific time.

Subconscious Mind: Goals

Your subconscious mind has no concept of time. It only functions in the present. Therefore when you communicate with your subconscious mind you will do so in the form of an affirmation. A goal for your conscious mind written as: "I weigh 155 pounds on x date," would become an affirmation to your subconscious mind that you would repeat as: "I weigh 155 pounds." The only difference is that you don't put a date on it. You relay this desire to your subconscious mind and it will find the shortest route to your goal.

You put the date on your goal for your conscious mind so that it becomes a believable goal and a target. This aligns the believability your conscious mind needs to the positive, emotional feeling that fuels your subconscious mind.

As noted earlier, our subconscious mind is our success tool, and unfortunately we were never taught how to use it effectively. If you wish to eliminate a bad habit it is imperative to write your goal in a positive/positive way.

Your goal must be positive because your subconscious mind cannot process a negative

---

* You will not be asked to begin the physical process of weight loss until the first day of week three.

---

command. It is only receptive to a positive, present tense statement.

STEP 8 – According to the above guidelines, write down a goal that you know you can achieve by the end of this course,* and a second goal (or lifestyle) that you would like to achieve at some future point following the conclusion of this course.

That's your step for day eight. Continue visualizing yourself as you really want to be. Make sure you're seeing that "perfect-body-picture" with your face on it as often as possible.

JOURNAL ENTRY

I'm the best reason in the world to change ... so I'll change!

Keys to Setting My Goals:
1. It must be something I desire.
2. It must be clear, specific, positive and present tense.
3. It must be believable, achievable and measurable.

EXAMPLES OF SOME POSSIBLE COURSE GOALS:
- I weigh _____ pounds on _____ date (Day 29).
- I drink the daily recommended amount of water.
- I choose lower-fat foods whenever possible.
- I found several easy ways to reduce my daily caloric intake.
- I go for regular walks.
- I consume _____ servings of fruit and vegetables each day.
- I do some kind of regular exercise.
- I begin each day with breakfast.
- I eat regular healthy meals and snacks. I don't allow myself to get hungry.

My goal for this course is: _____

_____

_____

_____

_____

My affirmation for my subconscious mind is:_____

_____

_____

_____

EXAMPLES OF SOME POSSIBLE LIFETIME GOALS

Lifetime Goal:

- I enjoy my life at my perfect weight of _____.
- I enjoy food more than ever. I eat what I choose to eat and I still maintain my perfect weight.
- I lost my excess weight, and now I maintain my perfect weight effortlessly.

My long-term weight/health goal for the way I will live my life is: _____

_____

_____

DAY EIGHT – P.M. MESSAGE

Give yourself a hearty congratulations. Writing down your goal is a huge step to its attainment.

Remember: Everyone has an image of himself, but feeling fat or ugly or sickly interferes with the body's translation of the desired image. Picture yourself as an image of health.

Try to visualize yourself doing something you enjoy, (walking along a beach, playing tennis, getting into a new outfit) at exactly the size and physical shape you desire ... just before you go to sleep.

See you tomorrow!

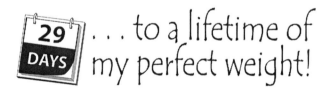

DAY NINE
I'm the best reason in the world to change ... so I'll change!

DAY NINE – A.M.

Nobody plans to fail, but many people fail because they failed to plan.

This week is about planning for action.

Yesterday you set your goals. Today you will begin to think of small questions that you could ask yourself that will help you achieve your goal. When you ask your brain small questions, you engage it. It *will* give you answers. Be patient. Asking small questions will also not disturb your amygdala. We don't want to bother waking up that part of your brain. Let's let sleeping dogs lie!

In *29 Days ... to a habit you want!* we talked about your *Reticular Activating System* or your RAS. Every single impulse, whether derived from thought, touch, taste, smell, seeing or hearing, first passes through your RAS.

The RAS then sends signals to the proper area of your brain for interpretation. When something important is on your RAS, it sends a signal to the conscious level for your immediate attention.

If you begin to ask the same question over and over, your brain (RAS) will begin paying attention and subsequently it will begin to create answers.

Begin to ask yourself some questions that could help you achieve a goal of losing let's say 500 calories a day. On day four, Step 4 we said that by losing just 500 calories a day, in six months you would lose more than twenty pounds without any physical exertion whatsoever!

STEP 9 – There is nothing that you have to do on a physical level today. Today's step is to notice your habits (which you're very familiar with by now) and ask yourself what small thing you could do to begin removing a few calories from your daily intake. This could be in the form of consuming less, or burning more (exercise), or a combination of both.

JOURNAL ENTRY

I'm the best reason in the world to change ... so I'll change!

What small steps could I take that would lead to achieving my lifetime goal of living my perfect weight?

Sample Questions you might ask your brain:
1. **What is one small thing I could do that would eliminate a few calories each day?**
2. **What could I do to get myself to drink more water each day?**
3. **What small thing could I do that would lead to some kind of regular exercise?**

1. _____

2. _____

3. _____

The answers you get back may surprise you. Let's suppose that you enjoy a morning coffee with two sugars? What if you put the two sugars in your coffee – minus a few grains? What if you did the same each day, removing just a few tiny grains so that within three or four months you were down to enjoying the same coffee with only one sugar? How much difference would that make over a period of time? The reduction would be so small you wouldn't taste the difference. In fact, removing such a small amount of sugar would actually be a fun daily challenge.

Keep asking your brain for answers. Make this a team effort, you and your subconscious mind. Once your subconscious is on board, you couldn't ask for a better ally.

What else could you do?

If you regularly park in a large parking lot each day, how about parking one car space further each day so that before long, you were getting some meaningful exercise?

Suppose you enjoy a snack of popcorn or potato chips on a regular basis. Rather than eat your snack out of a bag, perhaps you could put it into a bowl and then put a small portion of chips or popcorn back into the bag. This action will play a huge role in your subconscious conditioning.

If you were to do this over a period of time, you may be surprised to find that a smaller quantity of the same snack will not only be just as satisfying, but the self-confidence and feelings of inner strength that action will generate will be practically intoxicating!

What else could I do? _____

_____

_____

_____

_____

Remember, you want to create something that is <u>so easy</u> that there is no chance of alarming your amygdala. We'll keep that "puppy" fast asleep!

> Patience and perseverance are key!

DAY NINE – P.M. MESSAGE

You're doing great! Give yourself a pat on the back for another day of focus. If you already have some simple ideas that will reduce your caloric intake, that's fantastic. If you haven't thought of anything yet that's okay, your brain will work on it so long as you keep the question alive. Just make sure your brain knows you want an answer by asking for an answer periodically throughout your day.

You are making great headway. Stay the course!

When you go to bed this evening, and just before you go to sleep, say to yourself: "I like my new attitude" or "I'm proud of my new weight and health." Say this as you visualize yourself looking just like you do in the picture you cut out in STEP 3.

See you tomorrow!

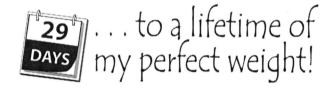

Portion Distortion .. the Hidden Culprit to Weight Gain

How much should we eat? One of the biggest hurdles to weight control is confusion about serving sizes. Years ago, a serving of french fries or soda pop was a fraction of what it is today. One doesn't need to look too far to see people drinking jumbo containers of pop the size of people's heads! In fact, a family of four could be sustained on some of the extra-large individual-sized servings advertised by restaurants and fast-food outlets. From sandwiches, to coffee to a plate of spaghetti, serving sizes are all out of proportion to our actual needs. The size of today's portions are a mirror reflection of today's waist-lines.

Since many people find it difficult to keep track of calories, we're going to give you some suggested serving sizes as an alternative to determine the "proper" amount to eat.

Recommended Serving Sizes

It is important to understand portion sizes in order to meet your nutrition require-ments while maintaining a healthy diet. Often, the portions we eat are bigger than we think and are also larger than the standard portions that are recom-mended .

Grains
1 cup of rice or pasta/cereal = fist
1cup of cereal flakes = fist
1 pancake = CD
1 slice of bread = cassette tape
1 piece of cornbread = bar of soap
1 cup of mashed potatoes/broccoli = fist
Nuts, 1 ounce = handful

Meats & Alternatives
3 oz meat, poultry, fish = deck of playing cards
2 tbsp of peanut butter = golf ball/ping pong ball
1 tsp of dressing, oil, butter, or
    cream cheese = top joint of thumb

Fruits & Vegetables
1 fruit/veggie = Tennis ball/baseball
½ cup canned fruit = light bulb
1 baked potato = computer mouse
1 cup of salad greens = baseball
¼ cup of raisins = large egg

Dairy and Cheese
1 tsp. margarine/spreads = 1 dice
1 oz cheese = 4 stacked dice
1 cup of milk = tennis ball
½ cup of ice cream = tennis ball
¾ cup yogurt = tennis ball

DAY TEN
I'm the best reason in the world to change ... so I'll change!

DAY TEN – A.M.

Welcome to day ten. You're doing great!

Yesterday we talked about asking your brain to supply you with some small, easy-to-accomplish ideas that would eliminate a few calories each day. If you ask a question often enough, your brain will turn it over and come up with some surprisingly interesting answers.

Remember: Always ask positive questions. Never, never, never ask a negative question like "Why can't I do this?" or "Why can't I stop doing that?"

Asking small positive questions can be a powerful habit within a habit. Asking questions will throw your brain into creativity. Your brain will have fun with this ... like solving a crossword puzzle or a riddle.

STEP 10 – Today is a continuation of yesterday. Keep prodding your brain to give you some fun and interesting answers. It will deliver. Just keep asking.

Remember: We want suggestions that will be so small they may seem too trivial to matter. We know better. Trivial is good. Small, continuous steps over a short period of time can produce miraculous results.

You may be familiar with the following test, and if you are, it's a great reminder. If you're not, you may find it quite surprising. The new thoughts and neuron patterns that you're creating are not unlike this example.

Let's suppose your goal is to accumulate as much money as possible in the next twenty-nine days. As you're contemplating the most effective way to go about it, the telephone rings. The voice on the other end of the line is none other than your rich, eccentric uncle. He says he's just aching to get rid of some extra money and in order to do so he's going to give some to you. He offers to give you one of two different amounts – your choice.

The first offer is an outright gift of $100,000 or the second offer is that he will give you 1¢ the first day, 2¢ the second day, 4¢ the third day, 8¢ the fourth day and so on, doubling the amount each day for exactly twenty-nine days.

Now remember, your goal was to accumulate as much money as possible in the next twenty-nine days. Bearing that in mind, which option would you choose; the first offer of a flat $100,000, or the second offer of a penny the first day two cents the second day and so on doubling the amount each day for the next twenty-nine days?

We know what the first offer will be worth at the end of twenty-nine days … obviously $100,000.

If you chose the second offer, by day ten you would have accumulated $5.12. Now which offer do you think is the best one to take? By day twenty you would be at the "princely" sum of $5,242.88. Change your mind yet? By day twenty-three you'll be at $20,971.52. By now you must think that the best choice is the first choice right? Surprisingly the wisest choice is the *second* offer. If you chose option two, on day twenty-nine your uncle would give you … $2,684,354.56!

That is the power you're generating by continually laying down new neuron tracks. Just like starting with a penny and doubling it day after day, it may not seem like much is happening at first, but stay the course! Great forces are happening. Great things are accumulating.

The most powerful force in the universe is compound interest.
~ Albert Einstein

JOURNAL ENTRY

I'm the best reason in the world to change ... so I'll change!

What small steps could I take that would lead to achieving my lifetime goal of living my perfect weight?

Sample questions you might ask your brain:

1. What is one small thing I could do that would eliminate a few calories each day?
2. What could I do to get myself to drink more water each day?
3. What small thing could I do that would lead to some very nominal exercise?

1. _____

    _____

2. _____

3. _____

Keep asking your brain for answers. Make this a team effort, you and your subconscious mind. Once your subconscious is on board, you couldn't ask for a better ally.

What else could I do? _____

_____

_____

I recently had my annual physical examination,
which I get once every seven years, and when the nurse weighed me,
I was shocked to discover how much stronger
the Earth's gravitational pull has become since 1990.
~ Dave Barry ~

DAY TEN – P.M. MESSAGE

Congratulations for another day of focus and being aware. You may already have an idea or two of how you might shave off a few daily calories. If not, be patient. Your amazing brain will deliver.

Did You Know?

We often rely on labels to count fat, calories and salt. When a label on a package says 200 calories, it does not necessarily mean that the food or drink inside the container amounts to 200 calories. What it will inevitably say is that it contains 200 calories "per serving," or rather, what the company claims is a serving. If the serving size is extra small, we may unknowingly be eating three times the amount of calories, fat and salt than we thought.

A box of macaroni and cheese (which many people consume in a single serving) gives out the salt, fat and calorie count, but it's based on ¼ of a serving. How often have you seen four people share a single box of "Macaroni and Cheese"?

In the early 1990s the U.S. Government decided to set a standard form of measurement. They had the food industry test, weigh and measure 139 different types of food. The government then determined the amount each of us would customarily eat, and set a size for each serving. The "solution" created new issues – their serving suggestions were ridiculously small. This allows the food companies to suggest their food is less fattening than it really is.

Read the information on the next four pages carefully. Next time your shopping or preparing a meal, take a moment and check out some labels. You may want to pay particular attention to portion size.

Don't forget to visualize yourself doing one activity at your desired weight. Try to involve all your senses. If you're walking along the beach in a bathing suit, feel the warm sand, hear the waves breaking on shore, smell the scents from the sea and the nearby vendors. Feel the lightness and aliveness of your body. Drive these thoughts deep into your mind. Try and visualize this scene for a few moments just before you go to sleep.

Congratulations on another great day.

See you tomorrow!

How To Read a Label
Serving Size

The first place to start when reading a label is to understand the manufacturer's definition of serving size and the number of servings in the package.

Hold on to your can opener, this may be a shocker!

Serving size tells you the size of the portion the manufacturer used to calculate the calories and nutrient values that are written in the Nutrition Facts table.

On the right are the Nutrition Facts from a box of Macaroni and Cheese.

For example, a box of macaroni and cheese, that many people consider a single serving, is actually calculated to serve four! So if you eat a box by yourself, you would need to multiply by four to accurately calculate your consumption.

Nutrition Facts		
Per 1/4 box (50g)		
About 2/3 cup prepared		
Amount	Dry Mix	Prepared†
Calories	180	210
		% Daily Value
Fat 1.5g*	2%	7%
Saturated 0.5 g		
+Trans 0g	3%	6%
Cholesterol 5mg	2%	2%
Sodium 350 mg	15%	17%
Carbohydrate 36g	12%	12%
Fiber 1g	4%	4%
Sugars 6g		
Protein 7g		
Vitamin A	0%	6%
Vitamin C	0%	0%
Iron	10%	10%
Thiamine	35%	35%
Riboflavin	20%	25%
Folate	50%	50%
Vitamin B12	8%	15%
Phosphorus	15%	15%

* Amount in dry mix
† Prepared as per Sensible Solutions directions.

Sensible Solution CHEESE SAUCE
ADD 1 tbsp. (15ml) non-hydrogenated margarine, 1/3 cup (75ml) skim milk and the Cheese Sauce Mix to pasta. Stir until evenly coated.

The % Daily Value

This is particularly important because it tells you how much of a particular nutrient a food contains.

It's a helpful guide to determine if you need more or less of a nutrient. The % Daily Value is based on a 2,000 calorie daily diet (not 2,500 calories) on a scale of 0 to 100 according to the Recommended Daily Intake (RDI) for vitamins and minerals.

You, like most people, may not know how many calories you consume in a day. But you can still use the % DV as a frame of reference whether or not you consume more or less than 2,000 calories. If a food contains 20% sodium per serving, then by consuming one serving of that food (assuming you're on a 2,000 calorie per day diet) you have consumed 1/5th of your daily requirements.

Understanding the % Daily Value can be most helpful if you want to lower your sodium intake or increase your intake of a vitamin or fiber.

You will notice that there are no % Daily Values for sugar or protein. The reason there are no sugar values is because there are no recognized guidelines for the amount of sugar that should be consumed. As for protein, intakes are usually adequate for most North Americans.

Calories

Calories provide a measure of how much energy you get from a serving of this food. In order to maintain a healthy weight, it is important to balance the amount consumed with the amount burned.

Notice the † symbol next to the *prepared notice* and how it effects the calorie count. In this case one *prepared* serving (most people don't open a box of mac and cheese and start eating it dry) is still more than 210 calories unless you use the *Sensible Solution* listed at the bottom of the box. In order to limit *one serving* to 210 calories you need to use non-hydrogenated margarine and skim milk!

Fat

Fat represents the sum total of all fats contained in the product – including saturated and trans fats. Saturated fat is what your body uses to make cholesterol, which can build up and narrow your arteries, a heart condition known as atherosclerosis. Trans fats raise the levels of your bad cholesterol, increasing your risk for heart disease and stroke. There are no safe levels of trans fats. Eating too much fat, saturated fat, trans fat, cholesterol, or sodium may increase your risk of certain chronic diseases, like heart disease, some cancers, or high blood pressure.

Health experts recommend that you keep your intake of saturated fat, trans fat and cholesterol as low as possible as part of a nutritionally balanced diet. You should aim to limit processed trans fats to as little as 5% Daily Value. A healthy eating pattern includes 20% to 35% of your calories from fat. This would range from 45g to 105g per day. (Depending on your gender and needs.)

Cholesterol

Cholesterol is made by the body, but some comes from the foods we eat. According to health regulations, listing the % Daily Value for cholesterol is optional because, while it is a risk factor for heart disease, a reduction in saturated fat intake, will be accompanied by a reduction in cholesterol intake.

Sodium
Sodium listings on food packages are based on a Daily Value of 2,400 mg per day. Look for lower-sodium and salt-free products. A healthy recommendation is to consume no more than 2,300 mg a day, which is found in as little as 1 tsp. (5 ml) of salt. Sodium may increase blood pressure, the number one risk factor for stroke and a major risk factor for heart disease.

Carbohydrates
Carbohydrates are compounds found in bread, cereal, pasta, rice, vegetables and fruit, among other foods. In the Nutrient Facts table, carbohydrates include starches, fiber and sugar.

Fiber
Most Americans don't get enough dietary fiber, vitamin A, vitamin C, calcium, and iron in their diets. Eating enough of these nutrients can improve your health and help reduce the risk of some diseases and conditions. For example, getting enough calcium may reduce the risk of osteoporosis, a condition that results in brittle bones as one ages. Eating a diet high in dietary fiber promotes healthy bowel function. Additionally, a diet rich in fruits, vegetables, and grain products that contain dietary fiber, particularly soluble fiber, and low in saturated fat and cholesterol may reduce the risk of heart disease.

It's a good idea to look for foods that have a high % Daily Value for fiber. Most people get half the recommended fiber required, which is between 21g and 38g, depending on age and gender.

Protein
Protein is a compound found in animal products, nuts and legumes. On a daily basis, it is easy to eat enough protein to keep your body healthy, which is why a % Daily Value is not given for this nutrient. For good health, though, choose lean meats and remove the skin from chicken. Try beans, fish and soy more often.

Vitamin A
Vitamin A is important for healthy vision and bone growth.

Vitamin C
Vitamin C is found in many fruits and vegetables and is an important antioxidant.

Calcium

Calcium is essential to healthy bones and teeth. Look for products such as milk, yogurt and fortified soy beverages with a high % Daily Value.

Iron

Iron plays a key role in transporting oxygen around your body and the health of your cells. Lean meats, lower-fat dairy, beans, whole grains, fortified cereals and dark, leafy greens all contain iron.

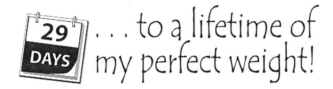

29 DAYS ... to a lifetime of my perfect weight!

DAY ELEVEN
I'm the best reason in the world to change ... so I'll change!

DAY ELEVEN – A.M.

Welcome, it's day eleven! You're doing great! You have every reason to be extremely proud of yourself.

This week's goal is to get mentally prepared to take real, physical action starting in week three. By the end of today you should have at least one or two ideas that you can use to begin altering your eating or exercise habits so that you can easily and painlessly eliminate a certain number of calories each day.

My concern is that today is day eleven and it's possible, just possible, that your inner-self (amygdala) is working overtime to plant seeds of doubt in your mind. It might be making suggestions such as: "This program won't work," or "It's been eleven days and I still haven't lost any weight," or, "Maybe I really like being the weight that I am," etc.

Remember all of the reasons why you want to lose weight. Refer back to the answers you wrote for day two's questions.

If this nagging self doubt is setting in, it shouldn't come as any surprise. We knew right from the outset that this would happen. Your amygdala does not want you to enter the action stage next week, and your inner-self is terrified of failure. The surest way to avoid failure is to avoid change of any kind.

Change is always frightening, but without change we simply cannot grow. Through this course you are asserting yourself, you are taking control of your own thoughts and actions. Growth doesn't have to be frightening. It can be fun and very rewarding. Remember, we're going to go slowly and steadily so that the change you make will be permanent. As you move further into this course you will begin to feel your inner self-confidence grow. You will begin to realize that these lifestyle changes will not only be easy, but they can become a habit that you can very comfortably live with. One success will build upon another ... like yesterday's example of starting with a penny and then doubling it each day for twenty-nine days. The results are magnificent!

A number of years ago, Louise Hay wrote a book entitled, *You Can Heal Your Life*. In that book she gave a wonderful example of the process of growth.

Think for a moment of a tomato plant. A healthy plant can have over a hundred tomatoes on it. In order to get this tomato plant with all these tomatoes on it, we need to start with a small dried seed. That seed doesn't look like a tomato plant. It sure doesn't taste like a tomato plant. If you didn't know for sure, you would not even believe it could be a tomato plant. However, let's say you plant this seed in fertile soil, and you water it and let the sun shine on it.

When the first little tiny shoot comes up, you don't stomp on it and say, "That's not a tomato plant." Rather, you look at it and say, "Oh boy! Here it comes." and you watch it grow with delight. In time, if you continue to water it and give it lots of sunshine and pull away any weeds, you might have a tomato plant with more than a hundred luscious tomatoes. It all began with that one tiny seed.

It is the same with creating a new experience for yourself. The soil in which you plant is in your subconscious mind.

The seed is the new affirmation. The whole new experience is in this tiny seed. You water it with affirmations. You let the sunshine of positive thoughts beam on it. You weed the garden by pulling out the negative thoughts that come up. And when you first see the tiniest little evidence, you don't stomp on it and say, "That's not enough!" Instead, you look at this first breakthrough and exclaim with glee, "Oh boy! Here it comes! It's working!"

Then you watch it grow and become your desire in manifestation.

STEP 11 — If you have an idea or two of things you might begin to do next week to work off a few calories each day then congratulations. Well done. If you haven't got any ideas, keep asking the question: "What small simple step(s) could I take to cut back 500* calories each day?"

Note: 500 calories is the target example we have chosen to use. This targeted amount will not only give you noticeable results each week (one pound) but it is also within the generally accepted guidelines of safe/healthy weight loss. With that being said, however, you may want to change that target amount depending on your individual comfort level and goals.

Remember: You want ideas that will be so small they may seem too trivial to matter. Small simple steps lead to giant results.

JOURNAL ENTRY

I'm the best reason in the world to change ... so I'll change!

What small steps could I take that would lead to achieving my lifetime goal of living my

perfect weight?

1. _____

2. _____

3. _____

The Hidden Power of Affirmations

Affirmations are one of the most effective ways of reprogramming your thoughts. Affirmations that you use over a period of time program your subconscious brain to help you make positive changes – especially the ones you are finding hard to do. Affirmations create DSP (Dendrite Spine Protuberances) connections in the brain that change the beliefs and attitudes that lead to changes in your behavior. (See Habit book page 26)

Remember, your subconscious brain takes every statement you send as literally real. Every time you repeat an affirmation, your subconscious brain forms new DSP connections. If you repeat them over a long enough period of time – say twenty-nine days – it will change your beliefs and subsequently your behavior.

Write out one very simple affirmation that you feel completely comfortable repeating.

For example:
- I'm making positive changes for my body.
- I'm willing to change by habits to be happy and healthy.
- I have a body I can be proud of.

- I'm happy with me and who I am.
- I have cut my caloric intake by xxx calories per day and I feel great about it.

My Affirmation: _____

Out of this affirmation will come the results you seek. Loving and approving of yourself will enable your body to begin to lose weight.

> *You will be a failure, until you impress the*
> *subconscious with the conviction you are a success.*
> *This is done by making an affirmation which "clicks."*
> *~ Florence Scovel Shinn*

Affirmations take a period of time to work, but when they do they are extremely powerful. Trust in the process, it's been proven to work.

DAY ELEVEN – P.M. MESSAGE

You are doing fantastic. Let's keep going!

Don't forget to visualize yourself doing some activity at your perfect weight. Write out your new affirmation every now and again. If you are the type of person who occasionally doodles, try writing out your affirmation instead. Writing affirmations is a dynamic technique because the written word has so much more power over our minds. When we write self-messages down we are reading them as we write them, so it's creating a double hit of positive psychological support for our actions.

Congratulations on another great day.

See you tomorrow!

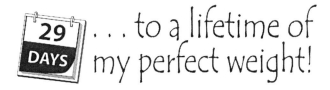

DAY TWELVE
I'm the best reason in the world to change ... so I'll change!

DAY TWELVE – A.M.

Can you believe it? It's day twelve already! You have shown all the qualities of patience, perseverance and the inner self-confidence that is so vital to permanent results. How do I know? You're here, that's all the proof necessary. If you stick with it, you *will* reach your goal of your ideal weight and it will happen sooner than you would have thought possible.

But there's better news. When you accomplish your goal of perfect weight, you're going to keep it off, painlessly and effortlessly for the rest of your life.

So let's look at some other concepts to losing weight and acquiring life-long health.

Next to air, water is the most important element to life on our planet. Water, or proper hydration, is your key to a lifetime of health and fitness.

Over the next three days, we are going to give you some reading material on the importance of water to your body. It's been broken up over three days because there's a fair bit of information to read, but also because this information should be thoroughly considered and absorbed. Up until now we have asked you to focus mainly on your food intake, but before we "dive" into week three, the *Action* week, it's crucial that you be aware of the role water plays in your health and weight.

STEP 12 – Today's step is to read the following information and give it some serious consideration and thought.

Water, Part 1: The Power of Water as a Weight-Loss Technique

There is indisputable scientific proof that drinking ordinary water is, bar none, the easiest way to fight fat and lose weight. In fact, the latest reports show water is nothing short of a metabolism-boosting, appetite-suppressing miracle. Some people may have a difficult time buying into this statement for one simple reason: you know lots of people who have the ever-present bottle of water and yet are still considerably overweight. So what's happening? Why the seeming contradiction?

Please note: This is not intended in any way to be construed as medical advice. As always, any issues or questions you have concerning your health should be discussed with your doctor.

You Must Drink It Right!

For everyone, except a few folks with rare health conditions, there are zero disadvantages to drinking water. There are only benefits, and lots of them. So again, how is it that some people drink water all day long and are still overweight? Two reasons. The first is that they're drinking tiny amounts throughout the day. To reap the biggest anti-fat benefits, which includes a thirty percent boost in metabolism and a fifteen percent reduction in appetite, you need to follow the following rules;

☞ **Have at least ten to sixteen ounces before each meal and snack.** When you drink this ten to sixteen ounces, don't sip it, drink it down. By consuming this much water you are certain that you'll have enough in your system at the time it is most beneficial.

☞ **Never allow yourself to get thirsty.** In addition to guzzling those ten or so ounces before eating, make sure you're drinking water throughout the day. If you are ever the slightest bit parched, you've dehydrated yourself. When we're dehydrated our body's systems, including metabolism, work up to fifty times less efficient.

☞ **Stave off hunger with water and save 100 calories per meal.** Research has shown that when we drink water with a meal, we automatically want fifteen percent fewer calories. That's about 100 calories less for each meal than when we drink soda, juice or milk. And water drinkers feel more full than people who skip water.

☞ **Water filters excess calories.** Drinking plenty of water allows food to flow through the intestinal tract quickly enough to reduce the number of calories that can be absorbed.

☞ **Water gives you a thirty percent metabolism boost.** The very latest proof shows that drinking ten to sixteen ounces of water increases calorie burn up to thirty percent for a full half-hour. You will also burn thirty percent more calories for all your waking hours.

☞ **Water helps break down more carbs.** When we drink water, our bodies use carbohydrate stores to fuel the increased calorie burn. So if pasta, bread or sugar are your downfall, drinking water will ensure that less of the pasta, bread and sugar you eat ends up being stored as fat!

☞ **Water helps break down more fat.** Fat cells are made of liquids and need proper levels of fluid to function. You simply cannot break down fat without plenty of water.

☞ **When you're well hydrated, you make all your body's systems – including metabolism – up to fifty times more efficient.**

So, for the rest of the day, try to note just how much water you tend to drink and when you normally drink it. If you don't like the taste of plain water add lemon, lime or a water flavoring packet.

Probably nothing in the world arouses more false hopes
than the first four hours of a diet.
~ Dan Bennett

JOURNAL ENTRY

I'm the best reason in the world to change ... so I'll change!

How often did I drink water today? _____

_____

What small step(s) could I take that would encourage me to drink more water? _____

_____

_____

_____

_____

Example:

- Keep a water bottle in my car.
- Begin a habit of starting my day with a bottle of water.
- Keep a bottle on my desk or work station.

DAY TWELVE – P.M. MESSAGE

I hope you were able to note the amount and times that you have traditionally been drinking water.

Don't forget to visualize yourself doing some activity at your perfect weight. Write out your new affirmation whenever you can. If you are the type of person who occasionally doodles, try writing out your affirmation instead.

Congratulations on another great day.

See you tomorrow!

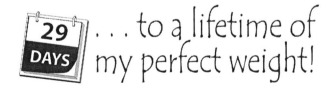 . . . to a lifetime of my perfect weight!

DAY THIRTEEN
I'm the best reason in the world to change ... so I'll change!

DAY THIRTEEN – A.M.

Hey, welcome back. You have been with us now for thirteen days, and rest assured, you have traveled far.

Today, we will continue with some further thoughts on water and its importance to your weight health and overall fitness.

STEP 13 – Today's step is further reading about the many benefits of water to your physical health and weight.

Please note: This is not intended in any way to be construed as medical advice. As always, any issues or questions you have concerning your health should be discussed with your doctor.

Water has been recommended by a large faction of the medical community as a preventative and cure for almost every ailment and malady imaginable. Its benefits for weight loss are indisputable and overwhelming!

The information has been broken up into three parts. Part Three will be continued tomorrow.

Water, Part 2: Overeating and Dehydration

Surprisingly enough, there is a very strong correlation between overeating and dehydration of the body.

In general there are two sensations related to eating; there is "hunger pain" and there is "thirst." Both sensations are felt in the same area and both are brought on by histamines. Ironically we will often confuse the two signals and think we are hungry when in fact we are really thirsty.

We frequently think a dry mouth is a sign that we are thirsty and we use that as our cue to drink fluids. In reality, by the time our mouths go dry we've reached an unhealthy state of dehydration, we've have reached the last stage of thirst. Have you ever noticed, after a heavy meal you are constantly thirsty? That's because the intake of solid foods help to dehydrate the body.

The best way to separate the sensation of thirst from the sensation of hunger is to plenty of water all day long and be sure to drink water *before* eating.

Our typical habit is to take food and then water. During the process of digestion the body uses up all the available free water. This can be a major cause of obesity. Here's why.

Obese people will often eat food to mistakenly satisfy their body's call for water. Food, like water, is converted to ATP. *[At the risk of having you shudder at the thought of a high school biology lesson, general writing etiquette requires that we give a brief definition of ATP.]*

> *Living things store energy mainly in the form of chemical bonds. Within your cells, energy is constantly moved around from one large molecule to another. To convert a food molecule to a muscle molecule requires adenosine triphosphate (ATP). ATP works like a rechargeable battery. When you eat, many complex chemical reactions occur, but in essence all you are doing is recharging your ATP, because everything you do, from walking to thinking, requires the immediate energy of ATP.*

Because this is absolutely crucial let's say it again. *Obese people will often eat food to mistakenly satisfy their body's call for water.* Food, like water, is converted to ATP. To the taste buds, food is much more satisfying than water. To satisfy the brain's need for ATP however, water is *infinitely* more effective, more efficient, and more desirable than food.

With food we can generate energy for brain function only from sugar. However, we will consume *five times more food* than the brain actually needs. Why? Only twenty percent of the blood's circulation goes to the brain. The other eighty percent, now laden with sugar, goes to the other organs - including fat cells that store the sugar in the form of fat. The more food we eat, the more sugar is converted to fat. Meanwhile back at the "brain ranch," all it wanted was a little water to generate hydroelectricity, a wonderfully clean, pure source of energy.

You may want to read the above explanation one more time!

Since many of us have erroneously programmed ourselves to confuse basic thirst for hunger, we have simply developed an undesirable habit (eating) to our body's cry for energy (read water). Dehydration is very often the *root cause* of obesity.

What's the solution? About thirty minutes before each meal, and two and a half hours after each meal, drink about sixteen ounces of water. Drinking sixteen ounces of water thirty minutes *before* eating, will help you to feel full and as a result, you will eat considerably less food at mealtime.

... Part three to be continued tomorrow.

JOURNAL ENTRY

I'm the best reason in the world to change ... so I'll change!

How often did I drink water today? _____

_____

What small step(s) could I take that would encourage me to drink more water? _____

_____

_____

_____

_____

_____

_____

DAY THIRTEEN – P.M. MESSAGE

This is now the second day of the information on the power of proper hydration. Please note your daily water habits.

How about a cool, wet tip?

A technique I used to train myself to drink water was this; I started the day with eight dimes in my left pocket. With each glass of water I drank I switched a dime from my left to my right pocket. At the end of the day the goal was to have all eight dimes in my right pocket. It worked. You'll be amazed how often you feel the dimes or you subconsciously put your hand in your pocket and say; "Oh yeah, I forgot all about drinking my water" ... and you'll fill up your water container and transfer another dime. If you find yourself forgetting, try the dime technique.

Did You Know? The best way to figure out how much fluid you should ingest daily, is to divide your body weight (in pounds) by two. That's the number of ounces of water you need daily. A normal glass is approximately eight ounces. i.e. If you weigh 150 pounds you need seventy-five ounces each day.

Can you think of how you might start to incorporate water into your daily regime so that it would become a healthy and pleasurable routine?

Congratulations on another great day.

See you tomorrow!

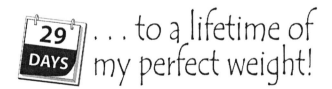

DAY FOURTEEN
I'm the best reason in the world to change ... so I'll change!

DAY FOURTEEN – A.M.

Hey, welcome back. Huge congratulations. After tonight you're halfway there. You have come a long way.

Today, is reward day. You have earned it and you deserve it.

Let's recap what we said a week ago about rewards.

Research shows that tangible rewards provide psychological motivation. Rewards are the easiest, most effective psychological motivators known.

When thinking of a reward, think small. Small rewards are a form of recognition rather than becoming an end in themselves.

> **Your reward should have the following two qualities:**
> 1. **It should be appropriate to your goal.**
> 2. **It should be free or inexpensive.**

What's an Appropriate Reward?
One that supports your goal.

What Small Reward Could You Give Yourself that Would be Free or Inexpensive?
Here are a few suggestions from last time: go see a movie, rent a movie, buy a paperback, call

a friend, enjoy some TV time, listen to a great piece of music, go for a walk, buy a magazine, take a long walk, enjoy a round of golf, or a game of tennis, etc. Think of something that you may not normally do and "DO IT!" Do something your really enjoy!

STEP 14 – Before you run off to enjoy your well earned reward, here's part three of the importance and benefits of water.

Yesterday we talked about the body's cry for water, and how we very often confuse the pangs of thirst with that of hunger. This "false read" causes us to eat instead of properly hydrating the body. Food is an inefficient way to supply the brain with energy, it uses only twenty percent, and the rest is stored as fat unless it's burned up through exercise or other energy consuming activities. We noted that drinking water thirty minutes before mealtimes and two and a half hours after mealtime will have a dramatic effect on our eating habits, patterns and quantities.

Part One of our discussion was about the power of water as a weight-loss technique and Part Two was about overeating and dehydration; today's lesson, Part Three, will be about water's role in helping you to shed the fat that's already stored. Just increasing your daily water intake will reduce some of your stored fat. In fact, you can lose as much as twelve pounds in three weeks by boosting your water intake.

Water, Part 3: The Magical Exlixir

Stored fat can only be broken down by specific chemical compounds. Certain enzymes break-down lumps of fat into smaller fatty acid particles that can be burned by muscles and the liver.

Water is the magical elixir that stimulates the nervous system and the adrenal secretion that leads to a gradual loss of stored fat and a dramatic reduction of excess weight.

Weight loss through proper hydration is more stable, permanent and reliable than any form of dieting and caloric intake. The most exciting part is that it is such a healthy and simple lifestyle incorporation that will have immediate and dramatic effects on your energy levels.

How does salt effect weight loss?

When the body becomes dehydrated and needs to increase its water reserves, it can only do so if salt is available to expand the extra-cellular water content of the body. A dehydrated body seeks salt through food. This search for salt is another bodily call that we often confuse for hunger, which results in overeating.

When the body is dehydrated, it automatically goes into emergency rationing. It is forced to allocate when and where water is delivered. Areas that are dry simply cannot function at their optimum levels. If certain vital organs and parts of the body are continually deprived of water they become susceptible to breakdown resulting in pain and eventually degenerative disease conditions.

Well, there you have it. As you can see from the last three days, there's a lot of magic in water. If you don't like drinking very much right now, just try it for two weeks. Use the dimes in your pocket as a reminder. The dramatic results will soon become addictive!

JOURNAL ENTRY

I'm the best reason in the world to change ... so I'll change!

Today is reward day. For my reward I gave myself: _____

_____

The second week is complete.
- Week one was about Awareness and Commitment. "I know I'm Committed to losing my excess weight."
- Week two was about further commitment and embedding those neurological tracks into a new, powerful way of thinking.

On day two you wrote in your responses to the following questions:
- Why do I want to lose weight?
- What will losing weight do for me?
- How will I feel if I could live my life at my desired weight?
- In what ways will my life be enhanced if I was to become my perfect weight?

Please go back and review your responses to these questions.

- Are you still in agreement with those answers? Are there any changes you would like to make?

Please take some time to do the following assignment. Write out a short paragraph, or even a one-line affirmation, that will help you overcome any negative thoughts or doubts about your success. Your amygdala will challenge you but only for a short time. Once it knows you are serious and that you won't be dissuaded from your goal, it will work to support you. That is when you know, and you know that you know, a smarter and healthier lifestyle will be yours, effortlessly, for the rest of your life.

You will not face a constant day in and day out battle of mental anguish and deprivation. If this were really the case, I would be the first to tell you to forget the whole thing because that is not living. That is not life. That is nothing but long, slow torture. Your new way of thinking is about happily adopting a new lifestyle. One that you are proud of, one you really enjoy. The best part is that the benefits are so plentiful that overeating will never be something you miss, it will be nothing but a bad memory.

Whenever I am tempted to discard my new way of living, the following statement will over-power any negativity and doubt. When I am challenged I will say:_____

_____

_____

_____

DAY FOURTEEN – P.M. MESSAGE

Way to go. You've completed two full weeks. You must be primed and ready to go.

As you know, when most people set goals, they start off at the action stage. The high rate of failure from New Year's resolutions, to diets, to spur-of-the-moment prom-ises of change are a testament to the problem of quick change and ignoring one's self-image. You are travelling a different path. You spent the first week building commitment and awareness. The second week you continued to build on your psychological commitment and you began to prepare yourself to face the challenges of the action stage.

You have laid the groundwork. You have prepared yourself mentally. Tomorrow we begin the action phase of shedding those unwanted pounds and embracing a lifestyle that will keep those pounds off permanently. This has nothing to do with willpower, these are simple changes that you will make. You're not looking for a quick fix, but in a very short time you will see enormous results. Remember Julie and Tom from

29 DAYS ... to a habit you want!? They achieved their goals in spectacular fashion, but they went about it like the Tortoise from the wonderful fable of *The Tortoise and the Hare*. "Slow and easy does it every time."

Now that you have prepared yourself mentally, achieving your goal is a fait accompli!

Congratulations on reaching the halfway mark. Tomorrow is an especially exciting day. See you then.

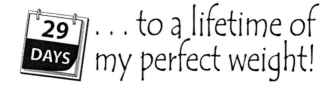

— <u>WEEK THREE</u> —

TAKING ACTION

DAY FIFTEEN
I'm on my way to permanent results.

DAY FIFTEEN – A.M.

Hey, welcome back. Today is the day we've been working toward since the beginning of this course. Up until now, you have been shedding your excess weight psychologically (creating new neuron tracks), but starting today you are finally ready to begin to shed them physically.

As we said in *29 Days ... to a habit you want!*, when most people decide to take on a new challenge they immediately dive into the action stage, which often results in failure. Spending the last two weeks creating awareness about your thinking, getting emotionally and mentally ready for the challenge has you *so well prepared* that the next steps will be relatively easy.

You have demonstrated the two ingredients necessary for success:
1. **Patience and perseverance — It's been two weeks and you're here with us every day.**
2. **Self-confidence — You took the task on and followed the daily steps. Without self-confidence we would all assume failure and not even bother to take on new challenges. With self-confidence we assume success.**

Since you're really ready for action, there's nothing your subconscious, inner-self-doubt, or amygdala can throw at you that can come as any surprise.

Should any doubts or resistance arise, just know that this is the last-ditch effort of your inner-self to resist change. Dismiss any negative self-talk and soldier on.

> Okay, let's take the first physical step to shedding that excess weight.

As you probably know by now there are a number of healthy ways to reduce your weight. In short, *you must burn more calories than you consume.* Over the next several days we're going to look at the four basic pillars to losing weight.

FOUR PILLARS OF WEIGHT REDUCTION:

1. Reducing the number of calories you eat
2. Proper consumption of water
3. Exercise
4. Increasing your metabolism

Your goal is to ask yourself, "What small change can I incorporate into my life that I can sustain for the rest of my life?" That is your key to permanent weight loss. If you have to spend the rest of your life counting calories and stressing over the fact that you lost weight and now you're worried sick about it coming back, then quite frankly you're on the wrong track.

You can incorporate one or several small changes from the above four pillars that will turn your weight struggle around for good. You can use just one of these methods or a combination of all four. If you choose not to exercise for example, then you will need to focus on one, or all three, of the other pillars – caloric intake, water consumption or metabolism.

We are going to give you a lot of useful information about calories, water, metabolism and exercise, and how the calories involved will directly relate to your weight. Since we don't want to overload you with information, we're going to give it to you over the next several days.

Today we will look at calories and food.

CALORIES

Most women need about 2,000 calories and men need about 2,500 calories per day to maintain their weight. To lose weight you need to create a calorie deficit by consuming fewer calories than you burn. If you eat 500 calories less than you need each day you'll lose weight at the rate of one pound a week. If you eat 1,000 calories less than you need each day you'll lose two pounds each week. Your body will have to turn to its fat stores to make up your calorie deficit.

The idea of losing 500 calories each day is not only a reasonable amount to reduce, but it's also an amount that is within healthy guidelines of permanent weight loss.

Remember, you are making some simple changes that will stay with you for life. If you find that something less than 500 calories is more suitable for you at this time then that's perfectly fine. *Our goal is lasting results.* That is how we measure success, and success breeds success. If you lost 200 calories each day for the next several weeks and slowly ratcheted that up to losing 300 and then 400 calories per day, you are totally on track. We're all different, and we all work in our own unique way. Steady, gentle, forward movement is the key.

You will be somewhere twelve months from now. Slow and steady progress will have you at your desired weight painlessly, effortlessly and *permanently!*

Remember to use self-talk, your personal affirmation and be sure to visualize yourself at your *perfect weight.*

Step 15 – Today is the first official day of calorie reduction.

Following are some suggestions that you might find useful toward living a lifetime of your *perfect weight.*

Reducing Fat - suggestions
- Use skim milk or low-fat milk and cheese
- Use water-packed tuna instead of oil-packed
- Choose lean cuts of meat
- Trim visible fat from meat
- Roast, bake, broil or grill meats and drain fat after cooking; don't fry
- Remove the skin from cooked poultry
- Use smaller portions of meat and stretch it by serving with grains and vegetables
- In a dip or sandwich filling, replace all or part with low fat or nonfat alternatives
- Serve peameal bacon instead of regular bacon
- Use vegetable or peanut oils instead of solid shortening
- Try substituting egg whites in recipes calling for whole eggs
- Use low-fat salad dressings

Reducing Calories
- Reduce size of servings/portions (measure of weigh food if you are unsure)
- Eat slowly, chew your food well. This allows you to realize you are full before you overeat

- Avoid automatically have second helpings unless it's a low-calorie vegetable or fruit
- Eat in a relaxed environment. It takes about 20 minutes after you begin eating for your mind to realize you are full.
- Avoid high sugar foods – read labels for words like high fructose corn syrup, dextrose, sucrose
- Use unsweetened canned fruit or fruit canned in its own juice when fresh fruit is not available
- Use slightly less sugar in your favorite recipes

Calories in Some Popular Food Items
- 1 tbsp vegetable oil - 117 calories
- 1 tbsp peanut oil - 119 calories
- 1 tbsp olive oil - 120 calories
- Medium banana – 94 calories
- Apple – 52 calories
- Medium grapefruit – 82 calories
- Large orange – 86 calories
- Regular Beer – 139 calories
- Light Beer – 103 calories
- 3.5 fl oz. white wine – 70 calories
- 3.5 fl oz. red wine – 74 calories
- Medium muffin – 170 calories
- Medium bagel – 289
- Domino's Cheese Pizza Classic/slice – 274 calories
- English Muffin cheese and sausage – 393 calories
- McDonald's chicken McGrill – 405 calories
- McDonald's Big Mac – 564 calories
- McDonald's Big Breakfast – 730 calories
- Taco Bell Bean Burrito – 404 calories
- Corn on the cob with butter – 155 calories
- Breakfast Bars including granola – 464 calories
- Fruit filled non-fat granola bar – 342
- Potato chips plain, salted 1 oz – 155 calories
- Air popped white popcorn, 1 cup 31 calories
- Coke, Root beer, can – 160 calories
- Diet pop – 0 calories

The preceding list could go on for many pages, but the purpose of this brief list is to give you a quick idea of the number of calories found in various foods and drinks. You may have found some of these numbers surprising.

If you happen to enjoy snacking on potato chips, for example, take your regular portion and put a few back in the bag. Or perhaps you could try substituting popcorn for chips. This can mean a substantial reduction in your daily caloric intake. If you do a search on the internet about calories found in foods, you can quickly find details on anything available on our planet.

Remember: Reducing 500 calories from your present consumption is our suggested goal. If your goal happens to be greater or lesser that is of course totally up to you.

JOURNAL ENTRY

I'm on my way to permanent results!

Tips and Suggestions toward Achieving Your Daily Caloric Reduction:

- Never let yourself get too hungry. You'll tend to overeat when your stomach's growling. Many of us can get caught up in whatever we're doing and miss our regular lunch. Then two hours later we end up gorging ourselves. To avoid this dilemma put some healthy snacks in your car or desk. Then if your sitting on the highway and feel those hunger pangs, you won't need to pay a visit to the "Chicken Colonel."

- Put some almonds, dried fruit, protein bars and a couple of water bottles in your car and desk, you'll be amazed how it will diminish the magnetic attraction of the golden arches!

- You might also try taking your regular-sized portions at mealtime and when your plate is as full as you would normally have it, take a small portion of something and put it back. Not only will this make a difference to the number of calories you consume, but it will have a tremendous psychological effect as well.

What can I start/stop doing in my life that will help me to achieve a negative daily caloric reduction? _____

_____

_____

_____

_____

The story goes that a husband and wife agreed to go on a diet together. They chose a diet that had a number of suggested recipes for easy weight loss. They were both excited and dedicated to their new goal. For several weeks they followed the daily diet plan and cooked their meals exactly as the recipes instructed, and when each meal was prepared they divided the portions exactly in half. They were soon telling all their friends about this fantastic new diet they discovered. It was too early to tell just how much weight they were losing but the beautiful part was that neither one of them ever felt the least bit hungry.

After two weeks of dutifully following the exact instructions, they began to notice that they hadn't lost any weight whatsoever. In fact, they may have even put a little extra weight on.

When they went back to double check the diet and recommended recipes they noticed the fine print. It read: "Serves 6."

DAY FIFTEEN – P.M. MESSAGE

Congratulations on your first day of burning more calories than you took in.

If you happen to fall short of your goal for today, do not beat yourself up, that's your inner-self's last gasp effort. Your inner-self wants you to get discouraged. It doesn't like change. Ignore it. There's always tomorrow to get back on track.

JOURNAL ENTRY

Today you have taken the first physical step in living a new life of health and your perfect weight. You are going to reach your goal, but remember, in every journey there are bumps along the way. Your journey will be no exception. The time may come when you have been systematically shedding a pound each week for a number of weeks. You've been praised. You have received endless compliments and encouragement and then gradually the excitement waned. This is the first "bump" in the road and how you handle it will be crucial to your permanent results. You may hit a plateau and seem to be stuck in your weight reduction. You may even notice that after months of success, for a couple of successive weeks you actually put a pound or two back on. This is precisely where most people slip-up. They've achieved a measure of success, they've lost a good portion of weight, and then for some inexplicable reason, they lost the slight "edge" that kept them on track. That will be the time to stand up and fight! Don't let all the work and accomplishment slip away.

You are going to write yourself a letter to read to the future. In the future when you hit the plateau, or you lose *the edge*, you are going to pull out this letter (whether it's on paper or on your personal online page) and read why you won't succumb to your old lifestyle and behavior. You are going to write yourself a powerful letter that will keep you from rationalizing the thoughts that living an unhealthy life and being overweight is not such a big deal. It is! If it weren't, if it didn't mean so much to you, then you wouldn't be at this moment in your life. It does matter!

Write yourself a powerful letter that will be your inspiration in time of need. This letter to your future will be a *powerful aid* that will help you obliterate any thoughts of returning to your old lifestyle. This letter will serve to blow those dangerous thoughts and rationalizations clear out of the water.

In your letter be sure to capture how you presently feel, physically, mentally and emotionally.

Before you write yourself that "Dear John" letter, here's an example of what you might say;

> *Dear John:*
>
> *I am writing to you from a previous lifetime, a time when you were unhappy with your weight, your health and your lifestyle. I write to you as your old self, a friend who is presently fed up with living a life of diets, binges, and periodic starvation. I am through with being at the beck-and-call of any whim that pops into my head. I'm through with responding to instant gratification.*
>
> *I know that as you read this letter you're recalling "the-good-old days," and thinking that stuffing your face with junk-food and being totally sedentary are part of the "pleasures of life." There are no good-old-days when it comes to being unhappy and feeling fat and overweight. John, I beg you, I implore you not to think these were good-old-days for even a moment.*
>
> *I have just started a new weight-loss program. I'm so excited about adopting a new lifestyle that I can effortlessly maintain. As I write you this letter I can hardly wait to break free and begin my new life of health and control.*
>
> *John you have lost x pounds and you have achieved it gradually and systematically. You have shown to yourself, your family and the world, that you are in control. You can live the rest of your life this way. If you've slipped don't get discouraged. Get back on track. You have created a new life. Overcome this temporary set-back and you're goal is all but achieved.*
>
> *Congratulations from me. I'm very proud of you for taking control and rededicating yourself to your life of perfect weight and health.*
>
> *Remember John, just hang in there. You've come so far, keep at it. Before long*

this new way of life will be the only one you know.
One day at a time. That's all it takes.

Love,

John

Okay, now it's your turn. Write yourself the atomic bomb, the secret weapon that will obliterate any doubts and frustrations if they come weeks or months from now. What can you write that will help you remember the place you are now, and how much you want to rid it from your life forever?

Dear _____

_____

_____

_____

_____

_____

_____

Love,

_____

Congratulations again and we'll see you tomorrow!

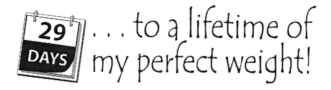

DAY SIXTEEN
I'm on my way to permanent results.

DAY SIXTEEN – A.M.

Welcome to day sixteen. You're making huge progress!

As you know by now there are four healthy ways to reduce your caloric intake and thus your weight:

1. Reducing the number of calories you eat
2. Proper consumption of water
3. Exercise
4. Increasing your metabolism

Yesterday we discussed calories. Today we are going to review water and its effects on weight reduction.

Step 16 – Today is a very easy "reading" day since it's basically a recap of the information from days twelve, thirteen and fourteen.

While reviewing today's information on water consumption
and proper hydration, continue to ask yourself:
"What small step could I take that would lead to
healthy hydration and weight reduction?"

Drink it Properly!

To reap the biggest anti-fat benefits of water – including a thirty percent metabolism boost and a newly discovered fifteen percent appetite reduction, you need to:

- Have ten to sixteen ounces before each meal or snack. Don't sip it. Drink it down!

- Never allow yourself to get thirsty. You don't need to worry about consuming a precise number of total ounces or cups each day but, in addition to those ten to sixteen ounces you down before eating, make sure you're drinking enough additional water so that you never feel the tiniest bit parched.

- When dehydrated, our body's systems – including metabolism – become up to fifty times less efficient.

- It's the anti-hunger way to save 104 calories per meal. When we drink water with a meal, we automatically want fifteen percent fewer calories – about 104 calories per meal – than when we drink soda, juice or milk. And water drinkers feel more full than folks who skip water.

- It filters excess calories. Drink enough water and food flows through the intestinal tract rapidly enough to reduce the number of calories that can be absorbed.

- It gives you a thirty percent metabolism boost. Drinking two cups of water increases calorie burn by thirty percent for thirty minutes, and you'll burn thirty percent more calories for all your waking hours!

- It helps break down more carbs. Drinking water helps our bodies use carbohydrate stores to fuel the increased calorie burn. So if pasta, bread or sugar are your downfall, drinking water will ensure that less of the pasta, bread and sugar you eat ends up stored as fat!

- It helps everyone break down more fat. Fat cells are made of liquids and need proper levels of fluid to function. You can't break down fat without plenty of water.

- When you're well hydrated, you make all your body's systems – including metabolism – up to fifty times more efficient.

So, for the rest of the day note just how much water you drink and when you normally drink it. Think of ways that you might incorporate more water into your life so that it can become a permanent part of your lifestyle!

If you don't like pure water, there are many flavor additives available or you may just enjoy a squeeze of lemon or lime.

JOURNAL ENTRY

I'm on my way to permanent results!

What small step can I take that will lead to healthy hydration and weight reduction?

DAY SIXTEEN – P.M. MESSAGE

Congratulations on your second day of calorie reduction. The most important thing to remember is that <u>slow and steady wins the race</u>, every time!

If you can make proper hydration a part of your life, you will not only see a big change in a short time, but your energy levels will soar!

Congratulations. Big changes are coming.

We'll see you tomorrow!

REMEMBER: TRY NOT TO LET YOURSELF GET HUNGRY!

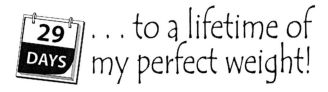

`29 DAYS` . . . to a lifetime of my perfect weight!

DAY SEVENTEEN
I'm on my way to permanent results.

DAY SEVENTEEN – A.M.

Welcome to day seventeen. Today is a review of the third pillar to reducing your weight.

We said that there are four healthy ways to reduce your weight:
1. Reducing the number of calories you eat
2. Proper consumption of water
3. Exercise
4. Increasing your metabolism

Today we will look at a few different types of exercise and their effect on caloric reduction.

Step 17 – Many people hear the word exercise and picture some poor soul getting out of bed at dawn and huffing and puffing up a steep incline only to drop from exhaustion at the top of the hill. Exercise, more often than not, has nothing to do with pushing yourself or having to get up at dawn. Everything you do uses calories, including sleeping, breathing and digesting food. Any physical activity in addition to what you normally do will use extra calories. Heck, just thinking about exercise can help burn excess fat!

You may recall in *29 DAYS ... to a habit you want!*, we talked about a *Harvard University* study published in the 2007 issue of *Psychological Science*.

The study tracked the health of eighty-four female room attendants working in seven different hotels, and found that those who recognized their work as exercise, experienced significant health benefits. It's a physically taxing job. Each woman scours a hotel room for twenty to thirty minutes, cleaning an average of fifteen rooms daily.

The women were separated into two groups; one learned how their work fulfilled the recommendations of daily activity levels while the other "control group" went about their work as usual. Although neither group changed its behaviors, the women who were conscious of their activity level experienced a significant drop in weight, blood pressure, body fat, waist-to-hip ratio and body mass index in just four weeks. The control group experienced no improvements despite engaging in the exact same physical activities.

The study illustrates how profoundly a person's attitude can affect ones physical well-being and by extension, anything else we are focused on.

Considering the above information, can you think of one small thing you might do that will lead to a little exercise that you can incorporate into your daily lifestyle? This needs to be something that is easy to assimilate and that you can do on a regular basis. Remember, we're only interested in lasting results.

Whatever idea you come up with, and if you ask your brain to come up with ideas, it will, the question to ask yourself is this: "Can I do this on a long-term basis?"

Following is a list of some activities and the calories they consume over a one-hour period.

ACTIVITY (ONE HOUR)	WEIGHT	130lbs	155lbs	190lbs
Aerobics, low		295	352	431
Bicycling, 10mph, leisure		236	281	345
Bowling		177	211	259
Child care: sitting/kneeling-dressing, feeding		172	211	259
Cooking or food preparation		148	176	216
Gardening, general		295	352	431
Golf, general		236	281	345
Mowing lawn, general		325	387	474
Raking lawn		236	281	345
Scrubbing floors, on hands and knees		325	387	474
Shoveling snow, by hand		354	422	518
Sweeping garage, sidewalk		236	281	345
Swimming, leisurely, general		354	422	518
Walk/run-playing with child(ren)-moderate		236	281	345
Walking, 3.0 mph, mod. Pace,walking dog		207	246	302

The previous examples are a way to help you think about all the activities we have in our day and how we might be able to work one or more of them into our lives.

Let's suppose you really enjoy gardening or taking care of your yard, but you put it off or hire someone else because you are too busy. Both of these activities, for example, not only can it be a great form of exercise and a way to burn extra calories, but it "could" also be a wonderful outdoor experience. If yard work isn't your idea of fun, that's perfectly fine, but the idea is to look for something that you can incorporate as a lifestyle habit.

Ask yourself what small things you can do on a regular basis that will bring some physical activity into your life. Think of things like parking farther away, taking one flight of stairs to the office, taking the dog for a walk, or considering where you might walk rather than drive.

Remember Julie in *29 DAYS ... to a habit you want!?* She wouldn't dream of exercising, she was just too busy. Then Julie started marching once each night for sixty seconds during a commercial break. Sounds ridiculous and pointless doesn't it? How can sixty seconds of marching contribute anything toward burning a significant number of calories? It can't. But it can form the basis of new ways of thinking. It can form new neuron tracks. With new thinking comes new beliefs in what's not only possible, but enjoyable. Julie's pointless sixty seconds of daily marching soon turned into full-time aerobics classes.

So again, if the thought of exercise has you breaking out into a cold sweat, ask yourself: "What small thing could I do that would introduce some form of exercise into my daily routine?"

JOURNAL ENTRY

I'm on my way to permanent results!

"What small thing could I do that would introduce some form of exercise into my daily routine?" _____

_____

_____

_____

DAY SEVENTEEN – P.M. MESSAGE

Next time you look in the mirror congratulate yourself for another great day, and for taking the time to ask those simple questions that will lead to a new life of health and fitness.

You're already on your third day of reducing your calorie intake. That's three days closer to achieving your goal of living your perfect weight. Your weight loss should never pit your willpower against your desires. This new life is not about teeth clenched deprivation. With that said however, you should also work to eliminate temptation.

- Don't buy unhealthy foods or frequent places that tempt your unwanted desires.
- Keep a bowl of fruit handy.
- Keep a bottle of water handy, and flavor with lemon or lime to make it more tasty.
- Keep dried fruit in your purse or car to avoid getting hungry.
- If bad weather keeps you indoors consider a treadmill or stationary bicycle.
- Watch TV or read while walking a treadmill or riding a stationary bicycle. If you enjoy the daily news or a favorite show, exercising while watching it can be a wonderful, lifelong routine.

Remember, ask your brain for a solution to a problem and it will give you the answer, guaranteed!

Just before you go to sleep tonight, picture what you'll look like in just 6 months from now. Will you be attending a reunion, a Christmas party, going for a walk along the beach? Whatever it may be, visualize yourself and how you'll look and feel.

See you tomorrow.

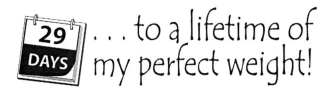
29 DAYS . . . to a lifetime of my perfect weight!

DAY EIGHTEEN
I'm on my way to permanent results.

DAY EIGHTEEN – A.M.

Welcome to day eighteen. Today is a review of the fourth pillar of weight reduction.

We said that there are four healthy ways to reduce your weight:
1. Reducing the number of calories you eat
2. Proper consumption of water/body hydration
3. Exercise
4. Increasing your metabolism

Step 16 – Today is a reading day and a continuation of daily action toward your caloric reduction.

While reading today's information on increasing your metabolism, ask yourself; "What small step(s) could I take that would lead to increasing my daily metabolism?"

What is Metabolism?

It's the rate at which your body burns calories. Very few people have a fast metabolism. Overweight people generally have a slow metabolism. A faster metabolism will enable you to lose more weight than your friend even if you both have the same activity level, diet and weight. Muscle, for example, burns more calories than fat, so the more muscle you have in relation to fat, the higher your resting metabolism. (Resting metabolism is the amount of energy required to keep your heart beating, your lungs breathing, your brain and liver functioning and your cells alive at complete rest.)

If you increase your metabolism (which most of us can) your body will begin to aggressively burn excess fat. With an increased metabolism, you have a powerful ally to easily lose excess weight and most importantly to sustain your *perfect weight*.

Your metabolic rate depends on the interaction between the number of calories you consume, the number of calories you burn while eating and exercising, and the calories you burn based on your individual genetic makeup.

Metabolism and Age

When we reach the ripe-old-age of about twenty-five, the average person's metabolic rate begins to decline between five and ten percent each decade, which means an adult will lose from twenty percent to forty percent over the course of their adult life span.

Research shows that people who maintain physical activity throughout their lifetime will only lose about .3 percent of their metabolic rate per decade. This relates to only a one to two percent drop over an active adult lifespan!

How to Increase Your Metabolism

Your metabolic efficiency begins with your digestion. Digestive enzymes break down food into nutrients that can be absorbed and assimilated by the body and then metabolically converted into energy for human use. Metabolic efficiency leads to permanent weight control, metabolic dysfunction is the principal cause of weight gain and obesity.

Your body can burn calories from protein, fat or carbs. Since your body is never wasteful, it will only burn fat when it needs energy.

This means exercise!

Exercise increases your metabolism in four ways:
1. Increasing oxygen consumption increases your metabolic rate.
2. Sustained muscular exertion accelerates the burning of fat and carbs.
3. Building muscle mass accelerates your metabolism at rest and at play.
4. Regular exercise improves your carbohydrate metabolism.

Muscle tissue uses more calories than fat tissue because it has a higher metabolic rate. Aerobic exercise, like walking, swimming or cycling, has the added bonus of speeding up your metabolism for four to eight hours after you stop exercising. Additional calories will be burned off long after you stop exercising.

Weight lifting, resistance or strength training, does not speed up your metabolism, but it does burn fat and increase your lean muscle mass which increases your resting metabolic rate. A combination of aerobic exercise and resistance training is best for optimal fat burning and metabolism boosting. Exercise in the morning and you will reap the benefits of a faster metabolism throughout the day. Exercise any time you can fit it into your day and you will burn fat away. If you exercise just a little more than usual you can speed up your metabolism and use up stored fat in the process.

Eat breakfast!

Breakfast is essential. Your body has been deprived of food throughout the night, therefore your metabolism has slowed. If the cells do not receive sufficient nutrients they will begin to function less efficiently on smaller amounts, and they will actually store more fat to use during these times of nutritional deprivation. Snacking on low-calorie healthy foods throughout the day will keep your metabolism revved up. Avoid eating late at night because your metabolism naturally slows down in the afternoon and evening, so eat a hearty breakfast. Consistency is important because your body's metabolism adapts to your current weight. If you have been dieting or skipping meals your body's metabolism slows down to compensate for the lack of nutrients. When lean people overeat their metabolism speeds up and when obese people diet their metabolism slows down. Such is life!

How to Keep Your Metabolism Humming

- Adding more muscle boosts your body's energy needs. Each extra pound of muscle you carry can burn up to fifty additional calories just to maintain itself.

- Your body will also burn twice as many calories digesting high-protein foods as it will burning foods that are high in carbs and fat.

- Adding just five to ten pounds of lean muscle mass will increase your "resting" metabolism by at least 100 calories each and every day.

- Obviously we can't exercise all the time. Fortunately your body needs extra energy at other times as well. One such time is after an exercise program. When your body burns extra calories following an intense exercise workout it's called "afterburn." This extra burn rate usually lasts from one to three hours, and in some cases even longer. If you alternate three minutes of moderate intensity with thirty seconds of high all-out energy you will burn an additional 100 calories during your afterburn.

- Each time you eat you stimulate your metabolism. Eating every two to three hours feeds muscles and starves fat. Skipping breakfast, having a quick bite at lunch and a huge dinner frightens your body into storing fat. A Georgia State University study shows people who eat every two to three hours have less body fat and faster metabolisms than those who eat only two or three meals per day.

- Always move when possible. That could even mean standing at times rather than sitting. Or it may mean walking rather than standing. Think about taking a walk to the other person's office, or taking the stairs rather than the elevator, or walk to the water cooler, walk to lunch rather than drive – anything that promotes movement helps nudge a sluggish metabolism and begins to burn that excess fat. If you've taken the kids to a soccer practice, walk around while you watch rather than sitting in the bleachers. A simple adjustment that will pay huge dividends.

> *Note: Frequent eating to lose weight and generate a faster metabolism doesn't mean you can eat Twinkies and potato chips throughout the day. Proper frequent eating is more like a mini-meal such as a protein or vegetables, nuts or fruit. Fiber is a non-digestible carbohydrate, but the body tries to break it down anyway, which uses up energy and boosts your metabolism at the same time.*

- Your metabolism is on slow when you sleep. Eating breakfast is a surefire way to wake it up when you wake up. It's important though to eat the right things. Many people eat only carbs which give your body and brain a glucose rush (sugar rush). Shortly after you'll experience a sugar crash (low blood sugar) and your metabolism slows to nothing. Your body goes into starvation mode, stops burning fat and starts storing everything as fat.

- Eat protein and fats with your carbs, the protein and fats slow the conversion of carbs into glucose, making them time-released and keeping your blood sugar levels stable. The more stable your blood sugar, the more energy you have and the more fat you burn.

So there you have some more "food" for thought.

JOURNAL ENTRY

I'm on my way to permanent results!

"What small thing could I do today, and each successive day that would increase my metabolism?" _____

_____

_____

_____

DAY EIGHTEEN – P.M. MESSAGE

Congratulations on another great day, and for continuing to ask yourself the question: "What small step could I take today that will lead to a life of health and fitness?"

Don't forget to visualize yourself at your perfect weight. Try to see yourself this way when you first wake up, and spend a few seconds visualizing yourself at your ideal weight just as you're going to sleep.

By now you probably realize how much your thinking has changed and how it's easily drawing you toward a permanently healthy lifestyle. You're building thought habits and patterns that will be with you for a lifetime.

You're doing great. Keep up!

See you tomorrow.

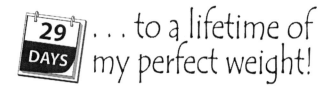

DAY NINETEEN
I'm on my way to permanent results.

DAY NINETEEN – A.M.

Welcome to day nineteen.

Have you noticed how much your thinking has changed in the last two weeks? Can you feel and see how changing your thoughts can elevate your awareness and confidence level? Can you see how simple changes do not rely on willpower? The changes you want, the changes that will lead to a lifetime of carefree body maintenance are found in simple, basic lifestyle changes. Burn a few extra calories here and there and before you know it you've achieved a lifetime of *your perfect weight.*

Change your perspective and you will change your life.

Step 19 – The next few days are going to be a combination of fortifying your thoughts about a better lifestyle through the incorporation of one or more of the pillars to weight loss.

Starting next week, week four, we are going to give you some esoteric ways to think about *how*, *why* and *when* you eat. You will be introduced to some really powerful and alternative ways to challenge your thinking about your eating habits.

You already have all the basic knowledge you need toward living a lifetime of your perfect weight. We spoke earlier about the power of affirmations. Please continue to jot them down in your journal when you have a moment. This will only take a few seconds each time. If you're a doodler this is a wonderful and empowering alternative. Jot down "I am healthy and fit, and I love my perfect weight," or "Nothing tastes better than being thin feels!" If you feel that these affirmations are hokey, find one that really resonates with you. This is an invaluable tool that can be used whenever you're tempted or whenever a negative thought pops up. A strong affirmation will instantly annihilate a negative or debilitating thought.

JOURNAL ENTRY

I'm on my way to permanent results!

What are some simple actions I can incorporate into my daily life that will help me to knock-off a few calories and gain my perfect health? _____

_____

_____

_____

DAY NINETEEN – P.M. MESSAGE

Kudos for giving yourself another great day, and for continuing to ask those simple questions that will lead to a new life of health and fitness.

Keep trying to visualize yourself at your ideal weight. Try to see yourself this way when you first wake up. Just as you're getting ready for sleep tonight, spend a few moments visualizing yourself at your perfect weight.

Whether you realize it or not, you are constantly enhancing your thoughts toward a permanently healthy lifestyle. You are building thought habits and patterns that will be with you for a lifetime.

See you tomorrow!

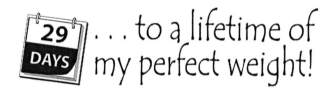

DAY TWENTY
I'm on my way to permanent results.

DAY TWENTY - A.M.

Welcome to day twenty. You've accomplished a great deal. You're here and you're making changes that will be with you for the rest of your life.

Did You Know?

It is estimated that less than half of the U.S. population has not read any creative literature in the past twelve months!

You are certainly in the "healthy" minority. Not only have you read the *29 DAYS ... habit* book, but you're here each and every day, making dramatic and permanent changes. And guess what else, tomorrow is day twenty-one. That means it's reward day. Think about what small but satisfying reward you can give yourself. You have certainly earned it!

Step 20 – Today you're going to continue to chip away at your extra weight. It won't be long before you can start to see and feel the results. When that happens you're really going to feel in control.

If you've ever been on a diet, do you remember what that felt like? Didn't it seem like a constant struggle? Didn't it feel like pushing a rock up a hill only to have it roll back when you neared the top? Wasn't it frustrating to know that the diet and its regulations were only a short-term fix, if that? Even if you weren't consciously aware of it, on a subconscious level you knew that when the diet ended you were at a dead end. Where would you go from there? You knew that it was never meant to be a lifelong solution.

What you've been doing so far is making those permanent changes and finding solutions that you can happily live with for the rest of your life. You are gently altering your course. You're making changes that are so slight they may seem pointless to someone else, but you know they're not. With continued faith in yourself and continued patience and perseverance you will be a different person six months from now. If you wish to lose thirty pounds, that goal is merely thirty weeks away. After that, all you need to do is maintain your intake. You can stop losing 500 calories a day. You can finish with the negative calorie intake and live the rest of your life in complete control of your eating and drinking habits. Is that exciting or what?!

Imagine a ship at sea. If that ship is supposed to go due south at 90 degrees for one thousand miles, and for some reason it alters its course by just one degree, it would be many miles from its original destination. That's what you're doing, you're altering your eating and drinking habits and behaviors by one degree. It won't appear like a lot today, but in six months from now you'll love that one degree change and you'll never slip back to your old thoughts and habits.

In his book, *Creating Health,* Deepak Chopra writes:

> *Everyone should eat a weight-controlling and healthful diet, not because he thinks it is good for him and will make him lose weight, but because he would honestly prefer not to eat anything else.*

> *So once again we are drawn to positive concepts like preference and enjoyment. They reflect attitudes that reside in the mind. I would like to emphasize that for most people being fat resides in the mind, and its cure will be in technologies that affect the mind and its basic outlook.*

> *A deeply held image of oneself as fat tends to keep that as the reality. The only effective therapy, then, is to try to change the set point through a change in mental self-image.*

Fortunately for you, you're visualizing yourself at your perfect weight. Seeing that picture of your ideal body with your face pasted on top is forming deep impressions in your subconscious.

Have a great day, and keep on chipping away at those excess calories!

JOURNAL ENTRY

I'm on my way to permanent results!

What are some simple actions I can incorporate into my daily life that will help me to knock-off a few calories and gain my perfect weight and health? Think about water, food, exercise and metabolism. _____

_____

_____

_____

DAY TWENTY – P.M. MESSAGE

Congratulations on another great day, and for continuing to ask those simple questions that will lead to a lifetime of health and fitness.

Did You Know?

There is no correlation between eating at night and gaining weight. But, people do gain weight eating late at night. Not because we metabolize food differently then, but because many people save their higher fat snacks like pop, chips, chocolate for the end of the day. Researchers say midnight snacking won't make you fatter simply because you eat it late at night. What makes you fatter is taking in more calories than you burn. A calorie is a calorie, no matter what time of day you consume it. As if you didn't know that by now!

See you tomorrow.

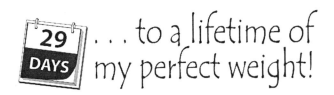 **29 DAYS** . . . to a lifetime of my perfect weight!

DAY TWENTY-ONE
I'm on my way to permanent results.

DAY TWENTY-ONE - A.M.

Can you believe it? You're seventy-five percent of the way there and today is reward day. You have come a very long way in the past three weeks!

You are so deserving of a reward that we no longer even need to mention why. I bet that by now, even your doubting inner-self will grudgingly go along with you in agreeing that you've not only earned your reward, but that you're going to reach and maintain your perfect weight.

STEP 21 – By now you're taking daily action steps toward reducing your excess weight. What a great day for removing just a little more! Meanwhile, be sure to give yourself a well deserved reward. Just make sure your reward is small, and will not conflict with your goal of weight loss.

Suggestion: How about taking a look at one of your favorite "decadent" recipes and find a way to "lighten" it up. I took many of my old stand-by recipes and substituted many ingredients to "lighten" them up - from beef stroganoff to fettucini to soups. Amazingly enough, by substituting low fat butter, or olive oil, reducing or eliminating salt and cutting the sugar quantity in half, I drastically reduced the caloric content and my family never noticed!

JOURNAL ENTRY

I'm on my way to permanent results!

Today is reward day. For my reward I gave myself: _____

_____

The third week is complete.

- Week One was about awareness and commitment. "I know I'm committed to losing my excess weight."

- Week Two was about further commitment and embedding those neurological tracks into a new and powerful way of thinking.

- Week Three was action week! You began to burn more calories than you consumed each day. You have found a number of easy ways to slowly adopt a new lifestyle.

I have incorporated the following actions in my daily routine that are systematically going to reduce my weight a little each day. Each of these changes are so simple that I can easily follow them for the rest of my life.

1. _____

2. _____

3. _____

4. _____

5. _____

6. _____

Albert Einstein discovered that a tiny amount of mass is equal to a huge amount of energy, which explains why, as Einstein himself so eloquently put it in a famous 1939 speech to the Physics Department at Princeton, "You have to exercise for a week to work off the thigh fat from a single Snickers."
~ Dave Barry ~

DAY TWENTY-ONE – P.M. MESSAGE

Way to go. Another great day!

You have successfully completed three full weeks. You are definitely in the minority when it comes to setting and achieving your goals. You have done things that most people couldn't imagine in their wildest dreams.

- ◇ You have set upon a course to lose excess weight – now by itself that may not be a great feat, but wait … there's more!
- ◇ You have taken the time and effort to mentally prepare yourself – now we're getting into much rarer territory … but wait, that's not all.
- ◇ You have written out your short-and long-term goals … this action puts you in such a small minority that you can probably host a worldwide written goals party in your back yard … but wait, there's even more that you have accomplished.
- ◇ You have written affirmations, practiced visualization and made deep changes in your subconscious thinking toward your health and eating habits. Wow, all this is me? Yep, and there'seven more..
- ◇ You have written yourself an inspirational letter.
- ◇ You have begun to physically reduce your caloric intake while armed with all the tools necessary to not only achieve your goal, but to make it a permanent part of your life!

You truly are a rare individual who should be very proud of all that you've accomplished!

Congratulations on such a successful journey. Let's keep on going!

See you tomorrow!

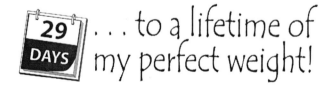

... to a lifetime of my perfect weight!

— <u>WEEK FOUR</u> —

STAYING THE COURSE

DAY TWENTY-TWO
Living my new lifestyle
of perfect health and weight!

DAY TWENTY-TWO - A.M.

Believe it or not, you're on the last leg of your *29 DAYS* journey. You should be seriously proud of yourself.

It's most likely that you're not at your desired weight … yet, but you have built the proper foundation of both awareness and thought that will take you to your goal. This week is about further embedding those neuron tracks of right-thinking deep into your subconscious mind to take you to twenty-nine days and beyond.

As we've said many times, you are the product of your thoughts. You have done everything necessary to lay those thought patterns that will keep you on the path of losing all the excess weight you desire. Remember the story of Tom? He was more than 150 pounds heavier than his desired weight and yet he *knew* he made it. How can that be? Because Tom saw himself, he really, really saw himself at his desired weight. From *that moment* it was never a question of *if* he would reach his goal, but only a matter of *when* he would reach his goal. Right now you are in the same place as Tom was. It's not a matter of *if* you're going to reach your desired weight, it's a matter of *when* you'll reach your desired weight.

By now you know in your heart of hearts, you're going to make it. You're going to reach your goal. You didn't go through this course for the sake of something to do. You stuck with it because you're committed to the outcome you desire. The desire of living a lifetime of your perfect weight.

If reaching your goal takes another month, six months or even more, that is not the issue. Your focus going forward is making sure that you continue a lifestyle that incorporates lasting change. You have made certain that you're not relying on the flimsy crutch of willpower. You have made small gentle changes that may not seem like much in the first week or two, but in two months the changes are big and beautiful.

Now that you've cut a new path toward your thoughts about food and why, when, and how much you eat, you will never be able to go back to your old way of thinking. Ever. Even if you were to slip temporarily, those thoughts of the right path will nag you until you return to what you know to be the right path. This is why your ultimate goal of living a life of your perfect weight is so certain. You have forever changed your thoughts.

The theme of the next eight days is entitled "Stay the Course." You have all the tools necessary. You have awareness, commitment, and continued action. This is now the most important week. If you've ever been on a diet and reached your desired result, then you have taken action. Since you have taken this course it can only mean that you didn't maintain your desired result. But don't let that bother you for even a moment because diets and that whole wacky lose-weight-quickly-world only lead you to a finite goal without any consideration of lifelong success. You are in a very different place now than you were when you reached a weight goal that resulted from a diet.

STEP 22 – Let's name today after the theme for the week. Today is "Stay the Course Day." Your goal for this week is two parts. The first part is to continue to put into action the process of losing the desired amount of daily calories. The second part is to be certain that the steps you have taken so far can be easily incorporated into your daily lifestyle. Give this a lot of consideration. If the steps you have taken can be incorporated into your daily lifestyle, then you have mastered the course and your desired weight will be reached and maintained for the rest of your life.

JOURNAL ENTRY

I love my new lifestyle of perfect health and weight!

What are some simple actions I have incorporated into my daily life that will help me to knock-off a few calories each day? _____

_____

_____

_____

Please note: If you haven't done anything in one or two of the categories, that is perfectly fine and entirely up to you.

REDUCING CALORIES - Each day I do the following things to reduce my daily caloric intake:

_____

_____

HYDRATING MY BODY- Each day I do the following things to make certain I drink the recommended daily amount of water:

_____

_____

_____

> *Remember: The best way to figure out how much fluid you should ingest daily, is to divide your body weight (in pounds) by two. That's the number of ounces of water you need daily. A typical glass is approximately eight ounces.*

EXERCISING MY BODY - Each day I do the following things to make certain I get some form of daily/weekly exercise: _____

_____

INCREASING MY METABOLISM - Each day I do the following things to increase my metabolism: _____

_____

_____

Have a great day, you slim, trim, healthy soul!

DAY TWENTY-TWO – P.M. MESSAGE

Way to go. Another great day!

You truly are a rare individual who resides in the uppermost echelons. I'm not being facetious. You are in a small minority of achievers. You should be very proud of all that you've accomplished!

Did You Know?

Calories are released at different rates. Fats are released at one rate, proteins at another. It takes a certain amount of calories to burn up each gram of protein. A good way to speed up the process of losing excess weight is to eat a high-protein diet.

Eating sugar on an empty stomach is seriously harmful to your weight loss goals since your body takes sugar in so quickly that it cannot be metabolized. As a result, it gets stored as fat. One third of the calories of protein are burned up just through the process of metabolizing protein.

Congratulations on coming so far. Let's keep on going!

See you tomorrow!

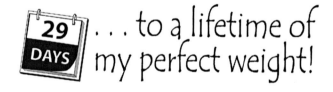

DAY TWENTY-THREE
Living my new lifestyle
of perfect health and weight!

DAY TWENTY-THREE - A.M.

Welcome to day twenty-three! Some studies say that it takes twenty-one days to form a habit, others say it takes twenty-eight, so depending on your take, you're already into your second day of your new habit or you're just five days away. In either case you have made some dramatic improvements and your life will never be the same.

STEP 23 – On day nineteen we said that we were going to give you a couple of esoteric techniques to think about how, why and when you eat. Today you will be introduced to an interesting way to consider your personal thought process when you're just about to eat. So today's step is in two parts: The first part is to continue to eliminate the designated number of calories you have chosen to reduce, and the second part is to consider the following information and how you might apply it to your life.

In his book, *Games People Play*, psychiatrist Eric Berne M.D. describes the three sets of ego states that each of us carry around inside of us. Each is active, and each will surface and express itself with a certain degree of regularity. In other words, everyone carries his "parents" around inside of him, and we each have an "adult" inside of us, and we all carry a "little boy" or "little girl" around inside of us all at the same time. The "adult ego" is educated, intelligent and rational. The "parent ego" is punitive and moralistic. The "child ego" wants everything and he wants it now.

One of these egos is always on stage, but either of the other two can assume the spotlight with a moment's notice. Talk about a potentially volatile situation! Now to be clear, you may know of a wise, gentle, elderly person who may never let that inner child ego take the stage, but just because you haven't witnessed it, does not mean it's not there. All of us have all three egos, but some of us may be able to suppress one or two of them much easier than others.

So how does this relate to eating and getting to our perfect weight?

When it comes to eating, the adult within us knows the difference between eating a Twinkie and eating a piece of fruit. The child ego within us couldn't care less about any consequences, and the parental ego will administer some sort of disciplinary action AFTER our child ego has eaten the Twinkie.

Here's the scenario. See if any of this is even remotely familiar.

One day you decide that you're going to take greater responsibility for your health. Being proactive your adult ego decides you're going to alter your diet by eating healthier foods and drastically cut back on junk-food. All is well until that feeling of hunger, or that certain emotion or whatever else might trigger your desire to eat, suddenly kicks in.

You may approach the refrigerator as an adult, but when you open the door your child ego sees a delicious cherry pie, a tray of brownies and a cold carton of chocolate milk. Instantaneously the child takes center stage. With the child in command you find yourself unwittingly wolfing down a generous sampling of all three – the pie, the brownies and the chocolate milk. The child in you, or any child for that matter, couldn't give a wit about calories, or excess weight. The cherry pie tastes 'sooo' good who could possibly care about anything else? In fact, of what possible importance could anything else be? The pie is in front of you. You like pie. So you eat pie. What's the problem?

As soon as you've had your fill of the pie, brownies and chocolate milk, the child leaves the stage. Since one of the three egos is always on, who do you suppose takes the spotlight now? If you guessed the parent ego you're absolutely right. The parent ego gets on stage and begins to rant and rave. "How could you be so stupid?" he screams at your child ego. "I thought you were going to try and lose weight?! I thought you agreed to eat properly? Now look what you've done. I cannot believe you are so weak. You've got no willpower! You're really a pathetic human being!"

So what's really going on here?

The parent ego is scolding the child ego. The adult left the moment the refrigerator door was opened. At this point either the child ego or the parent egos are in complete control which is nothing more than a replica of our very early childhood programming when we first learned many of our eating patterns and habits.

As we said earlier in *29 DAYS... to a habit you want*, the first thing we need to do to initiate a change in habit is to become aware of our thoughts and how these typical thought patterns have a way of unfolding. When we sit down to eat, we should try and be sure that it's our adult ego at the table not the child ego.

Do you doubt any of this?

Next time you sit down to eat with a few friends or family, or even better, at an all-you-can-eat buffet, if you're at all observant you can see people transform before your very eyes. Watch them load the food onto their plate, see how their pupils dilate, look at the intense concentration toward loading up on all the goodies available. Witness someone in that state and then tell yourself that that's not their child-ego running the show.

If you watch closely you'll see those childlike tendencies seize control of an otherwise austere person. Of course this doesn't happen to all people, since some people have trained their adult ego to be in control at mealtimes, but if they haven't, and the child ego is in charge, it's a fascinating process to watch. When an otherwise "in control" adult allows their child ego to take control at mealtimes, their language, physical gestures and entire demeanor will change during the initial eating period.

Now to finish the experience off, don't just notice the child-ego during dinner. Watch as the meal winds down and the reality of what happened kicks in. As the stomach becomes first satisfied, and then too full, you'll notice the parental ego coming to the fore. "Oh man, I think I overdid the over doing. I'm so stuffed. I wish I hadn't eaten all that food. That's the last time I do something stupid like that." And on and on it goes.

If you find yourself susceptible to handing over control to your child ego at mealtime, just your awareness alone can have a dramatic effect on the result and on which of your three egos takes control. How often have you taken too much food or eaten too quickly, and when you're finished eating you still feel yourself getting fuller and fuller and ever more uncomfortable? When that happens you know that you've overeaten and now it's too late. If only you had slowed down or taken a little less. If you can remember to bring your adult ego to the table, you will notice a vastly different outcome. You will actually enjoy your food so much more because it will come with a sense of appreciation and control as opposed to the actions of childlike gorging.

In order to give yourself the greatest chance to sit down at mealtime with your adult ego, try to avoid getting to the stage of being really hungry. Another very important point is to never ever eat a lot of sweets on an empty stomach. Whenever you put a lot of sweets into an empty stomach, the blood sugar shoots up, adrenaline and insulin pour out, and the blood sugar quickly drops. A rapid drop in blood sugar will bring back the sensations of hunger.

If you can remind yourself that it is your adult ego who is in control at mealtimes, and allow the adult ego to decide on "what" and "how much" you're going to eat, you will find mealtimes much more enjoyable. You will also feel pride that you can take control of a situation that may have seemed so out of control for many years.

JOURNAL ENTRY

I love my new lifestyle of perfect health and weight!

What are some simple actions I have incorporated into my daily life that are helping me to knock-off a few calories each day? _____

_____

_____

_____

We all have three egos: child, parent and adult. Did I notice my child ego commanding centre stage? If so what happened? _____

_____

_____

_____

_____

DAY TWENTY-THREE – P.M. MESSAGE

Congrats on another great day! Another notch in your belt, so to speak!

Did You Know?

A recent study, involving over 2,000 people, asked participants to use a variety of simple, and manageable changes to their daily diet, to see if they lost weight and felt better after one month.

The easiest and most successful techniques were:

⋄   Using a smaller plate: Those who down-sized their plates dropped over two pounds per month. They weren't using side-plates, but just a simple swap from a twelve-inch to ten-inch plate made that much difference. The smaller plate found people taking between fifteen and twenty percent less food. That's about 400 calories a day.

⋄   Another successful technique that produced a net loss of 2.1 pounds per month was to continue to eat all the same foods but "just enjoy" two or three bites rather than four or six. We are actually quite conditioned to be satisfied with the portions we take (assuming it's within reason).

Stay the Course.

See you tomorrow.

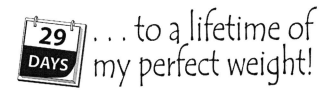

29 DAYS . . . to a lifetime of my perfect weight!

DAY TWENTY-FOUR
Living my new lifestyle
of perfect health and weight!

DAY TWENTY-FOUR - A.M.

Welcome to day twenty-four!

STEP 24 – Yesterday we introduced the three amigos – child, adult and parent egos. Today is an easy reading day because there's really nothing to read. But today is still very important, because it's another wonderful opportunity to reinforce your thoughts toward a lifetime of making the right eating choices. Along with being certain that your calories wind up on the negative side for another day, continue to consider the three *ego states* and the effect each has on our thoughts and behaviors. Does your adult ego stay or flee at mealtime? If it often flees, ask yourself this: "What small thing could I do to encourage my adult ego to take charge when I'm about to eat?" When you open your fridge, sit down to a meal, or reach for a snack, try to take note of where your adult ego is and where your child ego is.

JOURNAL ENTRY

I love my new lifestyle of perfect health and weight!

What are some simple actions I have incorporated into my daily life that are helping me to knock-off a few calories each day? _____

_____

_____

What small thing could I do to encourage my adult ego to take charge when I'm about to

eat? _____

_____

_____

DAY TWENTY-FOUR – P.M. MESSAGE

High five to you. You're moving right along. I hope you're still seeing that photo-
graph you cut out of the ideal body with your face on top. Be sure to continually
visualize yourself living at your ideal weight. See yourself at the beach six months
from now at your perfect weight. Continue to use positive affirmations. All these
techniques drive home those thoughts so that they're so deeply embedded into your
subconscious they become a permanent part of who you become.

Tomorrow we're going to give you another very cool "thought technique" that you
can use toward conquering traditional feelings of hunger. Stay the course. See you
tomorrow.

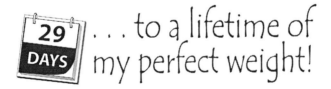

DAY TWENTY-FIVE
Living my new lifestyle
of perfect health and weight!

DAY TWENTY-FIVE - A.M.

Welcome to day twenty-five! Today you're going to be introduced to a very interesting way to think about hunger.

STEP 25 — Congratulations on another day of consuming negative calories, (consuming less than you burn). Today's information is rather unique. I think you'll really enjoy it.

In his eighth book *Healing and Recovery* internationally renowned psychiatrist Dr. David Hawkins, M.D., Ph.D., provides a weight loss technique that is wildly unique.* Dr. Hawkins claims it has worked for everyone who has tried it, including himself.

This technique is solely about controlling your thoughts toward hunger. I love Dr. Hawkins' technique, and I've used it with great success on a number of other areas (aches and pains) and it has absolutely worked for me.

Dr. Hawkin's concept is based on the fact that when it comes to hunger pangs we're all programmed to react much like Pavlov's dogs. Ivan Pavlov was a Soviet psychologist (1849–1936) who did a series of experiments on the phenomenon of "classical conditioning." In his experiments, Pavlov would strike a bell each time he fed his dogs and before long they began to associate the sound of the

> *Note: This technique may or may not be something you would like to try. Please consider this as just another tool in the drawer. There are many ways to achieve the desired weight you want, so if this method doesn't resonate with you that's perfectly fine.*

bell with food. After a while, the mere sound of the bell, at any time of the day or night, would cause the dogs to drool. Thus they were "conditioned."

We have been conditioned to respond like Pavlov's dogs toward the feeling of hunger. The minute we get that hunger sensation in our stomach, we have a natural tendency to label it as hunger and as a result we eat.

So here's the technique. Instead of labeling that feeling as hunger, you don't call it or name it anything. Instead, you go right into the sensation, into the inner experience of what you are actually feeling. The key concept is to let go of resisting those so-called hunger sensations. In fact you may even welcome them and ask for more. Mentally ask for the sensation to be even more intense. It's important that we don't label these sensations as hunger. As soon as we label something we give it existence and meaning. If we don't give it a name or label, it will have a tendency to quickly fade away.

The next time you get this sensation, which we normally label as hunger pains, just be willing to choose to be with the sensation, but do nothing about it. Let the experience run within you. Let that inner experience or sensation of whatever it is you're feeling just be. Just let it be. Some people may sense it in the stomach, and some may sense it as sort of a physical weakness. Whatever sensation is felt, don't name it, label it or talk about it. Just let it freely wander about in your mind; just let it be within you. You may even wish to move up to a higher plane of thought and say "I want even more of this sensation," of whatever it is that you are feeling.

We have all programmed ourselves to think that if I don't immediately address these hunger feelings the sensation will *not only* continue but it will magnify. In effect, that feeling of increasing intensity only results from resisting it. If you don't resist it, it quickly fizzles out.

The response of non-resistance is similar to the concept of martial arts. Force is never met with force. Resistance is never met with resistance. In fact, force is always redirected either harmlessly out of the way, or back onto the attacker. Picture a person running at you in an attempt to knock you down. In martial arts you would allow the attack to come at you and just before contact you could either step aside, or take the charge, curl to the ground on your back, and using your foot and leg hurl the attacker high and far behind you. The greater the force of the attack, the farther the attacker will fly. This is the same response that is called for with these so-called hunger feelings. Don't resist them. The greater the feeling, the quicker they will flee.

Most of us attempt to defeat the hunger sensations with willpower and resistance, but if we welcome the feelings, we will redirect them into nothingness. Just be with the feelings for just a few minutes and you will be surprised how quickly the sensation and feelings will dissipate. In fact, it will only take a few minutes and it will be completely gone.

So what's the point of all this? In effect, what you want to do is to break the cycle of feeling a certain feeling and then satisfying it with food. Responding to this feeling simply reinforces the cycle, which becomes a predictable behavior pattern. By sitting or lying down and really focusing on the sensation, you become the master of your thoughts. If you can sit through a little discomfort when that feeling arises, within a couple of days the feelings of hunger will completely disappear. This does not mean that we should stop eating for long periods of time or that we should even allow ourselves to get to this stage. The beauty of this little exercise is that it will clearly show you how you mistakenly react to a perceived sensation of being hungry.

The real key is what Dr. Hawkins calls "anticipatory eating." This means you never allow yourself to eat when you are hungry. For the first day or two, or even for the first week, (and it won't last any longer), you anticipate the periods when you normally feel that hunger sensation. (By now you're thoroughly aware of your basic patterns so this should be quite easy to do). So instead of waiting for that feeling, and then responding to it by eating, don't allow it to happen in the first place. Suppose you normally get the sensation of hunger around 6:30. Instead of waiting for that to happen, eat a sandwich at 5:30 when you're not yet feeling any sensation. You are now proactively breaking the cycle.

So here's the technique in a nutshell – eat when you are *not* hungry and *do not* eat when you are hungry and you will no longer experience hunger or appetite. Within a couple of days, and doing this a number of times, you can make the hunger sensation dwindle from a maximum of ten minutes to five minutes to very quickly lasting less than a few seconds. In just a few days you will be completely free of the conditioned response.

Remember: All you need do is allow that feeling to come up, be with it, even welcome it, and then wait until it rapidly runs out of steam. The way to break this cycle is to rise above it. By completely breaking the cycle you will find that appetite and hunger will disappear, and the experience of feeling hungry is gone forever.

What about the pleasures of food? This sounds like I'm giving up the enjoyment of eating.

Not so. In fact it's the exact opposite. If you can use and master this technique you will find that the appetite arises only out of the act of eating itself rather than anticipatory appetite.

Let's say that again – The enjoyment of eating arises out of the act of eating itself rather than anticipatory appetite.

You may sit down without feeling any hunger or appetite, but the moment you begin to eat, the pleasure of food is greater than it was in the previous model of - feel hunger and respond by eating food. If you break this conditioned program cycle, eating will no longer be associated with guilt. There will no longer be any association with calories or fear of gaining weight.

As you know, the philosophy of this course is about *increasing* pleasure, not denying it. If this technique called for diminishing one of life's most basic pleasures – the enjoyment of eating, it would be an exercise in futility. The entire exercise would not only be pointless but masochistic! So perish the thought that this will negate the pleasure and enjoyment of food, in fact you will experience the exact opposite of what you might expect. What you will find is that you not only have greater pleasure and enjoyment in eating, but you become the master of your thoughts and the proud owner of a body that is your perfect weight.

If you can break this, "feel-hunger-eat-food" cycle that you've been programmed with since childhood, you will experience an enormous sense of freedom. This technique does not rely on willpower. It relies on a willingness to use your positive, proactive energy.

Try it, you may find this ingenious technique to be the perfect solution. In fact, Dr. Hawkins warns that this relatively effortless system just described actually works so well that you may end up having a problem with being too thin.

JOURNAL ENTRY

I love my new lifestyle of perfect health and weight!

"I know that I always get hungry at this time of day."

From now on, I will not allow myself to get to the hungry stage. To make sure I don't get hungry, I will: _____

_____

_____

If by some chance I find that I forgot about food and I'm suddenly experiencing those sensations I will do the following technique until the feelings dissipate. I will: _____

_____

_____

_____

_____

DAY TWENTY-FIVE – P.M. MESSAGE

Four more days to day twenty-nine!

You're doing fabulous!

Did You Know? Foods high in carbohydrates have had a rough time in the past few years thanks to the success of low-carb diets such as the Atkins diet. But there's actually no proof that carb-rich foods are more likely to make us gain weight than any other food.

Ultimately, it's an excess of calories that makes us pile on the pounds – and it really doesn't matter where those extra calories come from. In fact, more often than not, it's the fat we add to carbs that boosts the calorie content, such as butter on toast, creamy sauces with pasta and frying potatoes to make chips.

Basic Tips To Smaller Portions
- Try not to eat while being pre-occupied such as watching TV.
- If meals are more than four or five hours apart have a fruit, dried fruit or vegetable snack.
- If you're going to have a second helping try waiting about twenty minutes.
- Use smaller plates and bowls. People who down-sized their plates dropped over two pounds per month simply from swapping a twelve-inch plate to a ten-inch plate.
- To get your metabolism up and revving for the day eat within at least two hours of waking up.

- Try to load-up at meals by consuming extra vegetables or fruit.
- When eating snacks such as chips or ice cream try not to eat them out of the container. Put a small portion in a bowl and put the larger container away.
- You don't have to clean your plate. Overeating and scraping your plate clean because people in other countries may be starving doesn't make a lot of sense for anyone.
- Keep large bowls of food off your dinner table.
- Try to put the leftovers away before eating your meal.
- When you're eating out, doggy bag some of your extra-large portions.
- Use leftover meat for sandwiches
- When eating out calculate how much is enough before you start eating. Or you may ask the waiter to only bring half your serving on your plate and the other half goes straight into a doggy bag.

Stay the course.

See you tomorrow.

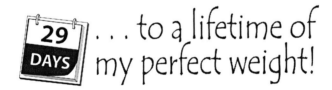

DAY TWENTY-SIX
Living my new lifestyle
of perfect health and weight!

DAY TWENTY-SIX - A.M.

Welcome to day twenty-six! Yesterday we introduced you to Dr. Hawkins and his thought technique on dealing with the sensations of hunger.

STEP 26 — Today's step is to knock off a few more calories. You're doing great, you should be very proud of yourself.

Did You Know?

It's a myth that we should only eat when we're hungry. We should aim to eat smaller meals and snacks every three to five hours to maintain top energy levels — and also to prevent you from overeating at your next meal.

Your body works best when it's receiving a steady supply of fuel. Eating regularly helps your body regulate blood-sugar levels and keeps your body burning calories instead of hoarding them. If you wait too long between meals, your blood-sugar levels could fall, causing you to crave a quick fix.

Dr. Yoni Freedhoff, an obesity specialist in Ottawa, advises that people should eat every two to three hours, ensuring minimums of calories per meal and snack and ensuring protein with all meals and snacks because protein is more satisfying.

"If you've ever gone to the supermarket hungry, you'll know that hunger makes decisions for us. Waiting until you're hungry to eat has to be one of the worst pieces of advice, because when you're hungry you make different choices."

JOURNAL ENTRY

I love my new lifestyle of perfect health and weight!

I have incorporated the following actions in my daily routine that are systematically reducing my weight a little each day. Each of these changes are so simple that I can easily follow them for the rest of my life.

1. _____

2. _____

3. _____

4. _____

5. _____

6. _____

DAY TWENTY-SIX – P.M. MESSAGE

High five to you. You're moving right along.

By now you can easily visualize your goal. THAT is also the way your subconscious mind is working as well. It can finally see that you won't be dissuaded from your goal. Knowing this, and knowing the new thought patterns you have created toward your health and weight, you will get the full support of your subconscious mind. All the answers you seek about the small steps you can take toward your goal will be answered.

Beware of Hitting a Weight Loss Plateau
There will likely come a time in your weight loss journey when you will feel like you've hit a plateau. You've been successfully removing a pound or so each week and then suddenly it seems as though the scale gets stuck, or your waistline reduction comes to a screeching halt. Hitting this plateau is perfectly normal. It's usually the result of paying a little less attention to the actions that got you as far as they did. When and if this happens, don't give up or get discouraged. Simply review the

behavior and patterns that you followed when the weight was coming off regularly and systematically.

How to Get Off the Plateau and Continue Toward Your Goal

- ◊ Review the steps that got you to the plateau.
- ◊ Keep a keen eye on portion sizes.
- ◊ Are you eating breakfast?
- ◊ Are you certain not to let yourself get hungry?
- ◊ Are you staying fully hydrated?
- ◊ Review the lessons on water and how it affects metabolism and helps dissolve fat.
- ◊ Have your exercising habits changed?
- ◊ Have you returned to snacking without being aware of the quantity?
- ◊ If you found that your diligence has slipped, get back on track and give yourself a reward.
- ◊ Have you gotten bored with any eating or exercise routine? If so, can you change it up to renew your desire, drive and interest?

Did You Know?

Often hailed as a healthy alternative to butter, margarines aren't always a better choice. To start with, ordinary margarines contain just as much fat and as many calories as butter and so offer no real slimming benefits. Worse still, they may also contain hydrogenated vegetable oils, which create trans fats – and these are thought to be as harmful to our heart health as saturates.

Stay the course.

See you tomorrow.

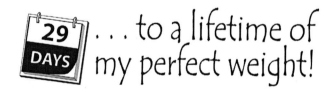

DAY TWENTY-SEVEN
Living my new lifestyle
of perfect health and weight!

DAY TWENTY-SEVEN - A.M.

Welcome to day twenty-seven!

STEP 27 – Today's step is to continue to live in the negative calorie zone.

JOURNAL ENTRY

I love my new lifestyle of perfect health and weight!

At this stage it's very important that you can answer <u>yes</u> to the following questions:

Am I comfortable with my physical progress so far? _____

Am I confident that if I continue my present daily lifestyle that I will lose my excess weight by
the date I have chosen? _____

Can I see myself living in this manner permanently? _____

If you answered yes to the above questions you are there. If you didn't answer yes to all of
the above questions please ask yourself this question:

What small thing could I do that would turn my answer from a <u>no</u> to a <u>yes</u>? _____

_____

DAY TWENTY-SEVEN – P.M. MESSAGE

Can you believe it? Day twenty-seven! You belong to a select group of people. You really have accomplished a great deal and you have proven to yourself that you have the metal to achieve whatever you desire. Congratulations!

Hitting the Weight Plateau

As we said yesterday evening, it's not unusual for people with long-term goals of healthy weight-loss and permanent life style change, to see their regular, weekly loss of a pound or so, come to a temporary halt. When it does, the manner in which you handle it can be the fork-in-the-road between lifelong success and a failed attempt. The first thing to know is that you have not hit a deadend. You have not reached the limit of your weight loss journey. What you have done is probably slip a minute amount in the four categories of weight loss; caloric intake, use of water, metabolism and exercise.

You may unwittingly be living at the level you will comfortably live at for the rest of your life. In other words you've slipped from being calorie negative to calorie neutral. Until you reach your desired weight, you have to maintain the daily negative caloric intake.

To get back on track toward shedding the last few pounds is often nothing more than a simple reevaluation. You can look at hitting this plateau as a point of discouragement or a fortunate opportunity to remind yourself of your lifelong goal of health and well-being. It's a wonderful occasion to recalibrate your thinking, actions and behavior to embrace the healthy new lifestyle you are dedicated to living.

It's All in How You Think

- ◇ Remind yourself that you are living a lifetime of health and well-being, not a temporary fad diet.
- ◇ Try changing something. A new exercise, a new snacking pattern (or not), find the rut, whatever it is, and climb out of it.
- ◇ Perhaps you should re-initiate the rewards program.
- ◇ Remember the value of patience and perseverance. Slowly but surely will get you there every time. Visualize yourself on the beach at your perfect weight. You know you can get there.
- ◇ Start the 29 DAYS program again to serve as a powerful reminder of the new life you chose to live.

◇   On day fifteen you wrote yourself a powerful letter for exactly this
occasion. Re-read it.
Remember the old lifestyle and how much you wanted to be rid of
it forever. Use this letter to get that edge back. That edge is the
slight difference between a lifetime of success or a failed attempt.

Did You Know?
Cereal bars might sound like a healthy alternative to chocolate but check the ingredients and you'll often find more than just oats, cereals, nuts and dried fruit.

It's true they're usually lower in fat than most bars of chocolate (unless they're
packed with nuts and seeds) but they often contain just as much sugar, which might
appear in the ingredients list as rice syrup, maltodextrin, glucose-fructose syrup, raw
cane sugar, fructose, honey, or a mixture of these.

But those aren't the flavors. That'd make too much sense.
Apple and pear, according to Dr. Phil, are body types the bars are made for.
Hey, I've got some advice. If you look like an apple or a pear, eat an apple or a pear!"
~ Lewis Black (On Dr. Phil's energy bars)

See you tomorrow!

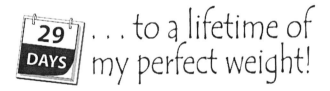

DAY TWENTY-EIGHT
Living my new lifestyle
of perfect health and weight!

DAY TWENTY-EIGHT - A.M.

Welcome to day twenty-eight! It's here again … reward day!

By now you know, and you know that you know, that you totally deserve a reward. You also know that the best reward is a small reward, because the reward is not the reason for doing what you do, it's just a really nice way to recognize and salute your achievements.

STEP 28 – Today's step is to continue to live in the negative calorie zone to *and* to give yourself your well deserved reward.

JOURNAL ENTRY

I love my new lifestyle of perfect health and weight!

Today is reward day. For my well deserved reward I gave myself: _____

_____

The fourth week is complete!

✓ Week one was about Awareness and Commitment. "I know I'm Committed to losing my excess weight."

✓ Week two was about further commitment and embedding those neurological tracks into a new and powerful way of thinking.

✓ Week three was action week! You began to burn more calories than you consumed each day. You have found a number of easy ways to slowly adopt a new lifestyle.

✓ Week four was about staying the course. You have made small, simple changes to your lifestyle that are minor enough not to upset your amygdala, but major enough to change your life in just a matter of months.

I have incorporated the following actions in my daily routine that are systematically going to reduce my weight a little each day. These changes are so simple I can easily live the rest of my life according to these new patterns and habits.

1. _____

2. _____

3. _____

4. _____

5. _____

6. _____

DAY TWENTY-EIGHT – P.M. MESSAGE

I hope you really enjoyed your reward today. You should be very proud of yourself. There can no longer be even the slightest chance of wondering if you'll achieve your perfect weight, the only question remaining now is <u>when</u>!

None of us are perfect, so don't even bother striving for perfection. Remember, everything you have been working for and striving toward is about adapting simple changes that will result in a new sustainable lifestyle for the rest of your life. If you should slip at any time, that is hardly reason to revert to an unhealthy lifestyle.

If you slip up, simply focus on the emotions, fears or anxieties that caused you to slip and deal with them. After all, we established quite some time ago that you are the master of your destiny and your fate.

See you tomorrow.

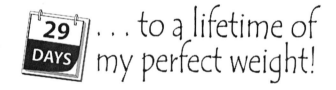

... to a lifetime of my perfect weight!

DAY TWENTY-NINE
Living my new lifestyle
of perfect health and weight!

DAY TWENTY-NINE - A.M.

You made it! You stuck with it all the way. You must be feeling very proud of yourself … and you should be.

STEP 29 – In *29 DAYS … to a habit you want!* and in this course, we stressed that living a life of your perfect weight wasn't about forcing yourself into a twenty-nine day timeline. The *29 DAYS* course was a matter of understanding your old thought patterns toward eating and health, and then using the rest of the course to overwrite those old patterns into ones that you desire. Your new thoughts aren't about depriving yourself of anything, they're about enjoying the steps you can take towards an enjoyable life of health and fitness.

On day eight you were asked to write out two goals: one was your goal for the rest of this course, and the other was a lifetime goal. I'm going to ask you to look at that lifetime goal, and make a slight adjustment. Very often when we think of a goal, it becomes a target, an end in itself – somewhat like a diet. As you know by now, your goal is not about living a life of deprivation and sacrifice, but rather living a life of making better choices and enjoying all the wonderful feelings and benefits of living your perfect weight for the rest of your life.

For these reasons why not change your lifetime goal from a goal to an *intention*? Goals represent a finish line, but intention represents achievement and mastery.

Intending to live your life a certain way is infinitely more powerful and lasting than setting a goal. You see, there really is no goal when it comes to a lifestyle because it's so much more than that. It becomes something that you are. It's an intention to live your life the way you choose to live it. Please review the lifetime goal you wrote down and reshape it as the way you intend to live the rest of your life.

JOURNAL ENTRY

I love my new lifestyle of perfect health and weight!

On day eight I wrote out my lifetime goal.

I now change my lifetime goal to my lifetime intention.

I intend to live the rest of my life by these principles.

From here forward, my long-term weight/health intention is to live my life in the following manner: _____

_____

_____

DAY TWENTY-NINE – P.M. MESSAGE

Wow! What can we say? You did it. You have passed with flying colors!

You have truly begun a new life. When you first started you probably couldn't imagine how you could easily and effortlessly achieve your goals. Now you know. The secret is patience and perseverance and small daily victories. Your new habits and ways of thinking are life sustainable. You have outgrown the childish notions of instantaneous, "I-want-it-now" results.

You should be extremely proud of yourself for all that you have accomplished. The only thing that stands between you and your goal is time - just a few months. Your new lifestyle will quite likely require a periodic checkup. Every so often make sure youre staying on track through the four pillars of maintaining a healthy lifestyle; calories, water, metabolism and exercise. Your aim is to adopt this new lifestyle as your natural lifestyle.

You are invited to sign-up for the *29 DAYS ... to your perfect weight* course as often as you wish. It's yours for life.

At this stage you won't have achieved your physical goal and desired weight, but you have achieved the must have first step ... you've changed your thoughts, attitudes and behaviors. Your old thoughts of eating, health, and lifestyle choices have been replaced by new thoughts of your own choosing. From here on in you are living your life with the unlimited power of intention. Your intention.

I want to thank you so much for participating. Congratulations for all that you've accomplished!

You really are special!

Good luck and long life!

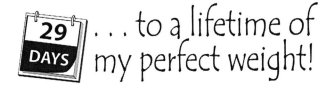

About the Authors

Michele Bertolin, has gone from fad diets, to health clubs to personal trainers, in fact, she has tried it all and nothing had a lasting effect on her weight.

Refusing to belief that she had to either wrestle with diets or live her life being overweight, she began her own research into the field. It wasn't long before she realized that most diets and weight-loss programs focused on the effect (the food we eat) rather than the cause (our thoughts, compulsions and habits).

With this new understanding Michele began to change her deepest thoughts and beliefs. Without compromising her gastronomic passion, she found an easy way to savor all of the foods she loved while systematically shedding unwanted pounds.

After several years of effortlessly living at her ideal weight, Michele developed her simple, straightforward strategy into the *29 DAYS … to your perfect weight* program.

Richard Fast, the author and creator of more than thirty toys, games, puzzles and books, has devoted the past twenty years to the research and development of the *29 DAYS* program(s).

He, like the rest of us, had always been told, "If you want to change your life just change your thoughts." That was the challenge.

Richard discovered that we *can* change our fundamental thoughts into desirable new habits by following the same cognitive procedure that we used to create our existing habits.

Richard's *29 DAYS* template for change uses proven scientific techniques, technology and online coaching, to guide you through a step-by-step process toward changing your thoughts and acquiring desirable new habits … permanently.

LaVergne, TN USA
16 June 2010
186368LV00003B/6/P